Occupational Health and Hygiene in Industries

Occupational Health and Hygiene in Industries

Raja Sekhar Mamillapalli

P. Visweswara Rao

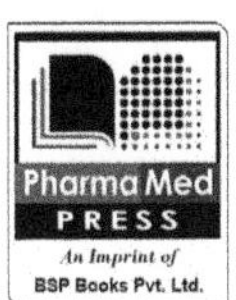

PharmaMed Press

An imprint of BSP Books Pvt. Ltd.

4-4-309/316, Giriraj Lane,

Sultan Bazar, Hyderabad - 500 095.

Occupational Health and Hygiene in Industries
***by* Raja Sekhar Mamillapalli and P. Visweswara Rao.**

Published by

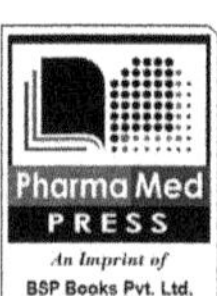

PharmaMed Press

An imprint of BSP Books Pvt. Ltd.

4-4-309/316, Giriraj Lane, Sultan Bazar, Hyderabad - 500 095.

Phone: 040-23445688; Fax: 91+40-23445611

E-mail: info@pharmamedpress.com

www.bspbooks.net/pharmamedpress.net

ISBN: 978-93-90211-36-4 (Hardbound)

....the arts men practice are various and diverse and from them may arise many diseases. Accordingly I have tried to unearth in the shops of craftsman, for these shops are schools whence one can depart with more precise knowledge whatever may appeal to the taste of investigators, and which is the main thing, to suggest medical precautions for the prevention and treatment of such diseases as usually affect the workers ...... a doctor.....should.....question ....carefully, ...what occupation does he follow ?

...........Ramazzini

Preface

Recent international surveys in Occupational Health have demonstrated the occurrence of a wide variety of health problems affecting the working populations, particularly in the developing world. Workers are increasingly exposed to new health hazards associated with industrialisation and mechanisation in agriculture, small scale industries, mining and construction as they are not equipped with essential protective measures against occupational health risks.

Over the past decades, there has been a considerable increase in the use of chemicals in industries. The industrial activities involving hazardous chemicals have the potential to cause occupational diseases, accidents, and pollution to the environment, if effective chemical safety measures are not observed. The indiscriminate, negligent handling of chemicals in work activities may be associated with the risk of occupational diseases. There is a growing need to create an effective control system in the processes involved and continuous care during manufacture, treatment of effluents, packaging, Storage, transportation, use and sale. This implies that the physician must be able to recognise work related illnesses so as to take appropriate action, not only to institute proper treatment, but to assure that patient care is coordinated with management of working environment by those in control so that recurrence of such illnesses may be prevented.

This book would be useful to Managements of Industrial establishments for scientific selection, placement, and statutory maintenance of personnel by pre-employment, periodical medical examinations for occupational health and safety in industries.

This book also provides comprehensive information not only to Industrial Medical and Safety officers but also to the students of Environmental Sciences, Industrial Hygiene, and Industrial safety courses.

-Authors

Contents

CHAPTER 1: Industrial Hygiene

CHAPTER 2: Personal Hygiene

CHAPTER 3: Chemical Hazards

CHAPTER 4: Personal Protective Equipment

CHAPTER 7: Occupational Health Hazard

CHAPTER 8: Fundamentals of First Aid

CHAPTER 1

Industrial Hygiene

1.1 History

There has been an awareness of industrial hygiene since antiquity. The environmental and its relation to worker health was recognised as early as fourth century BC when Hippocrates noted lead toxicity in the mining industry, in the first century AD, Pliny the Elder, a Roman scholar, perceived health risks to those working with zinc and sulphur. He devised a face mask made from an animal bladder to protect workers from exposures of copper miners to acid mists.

In **1713 Bernardino Ramazzini** published the first book that could be considered a complete treatise on occupational diseases, **De Morbis Artificum Diatriba**. From his own observations he accurately described scores of occupations, their hazards, and resulting diseases. Although he recommended some specific as well as general preventive measures (workers should cover their faces to avoid breathing dust), most of his control recommendations were therapeutic and curative. While he had a vast knowledge of the literature of his time, it has been suggested that many of the works he cited were of questionable scientific validity, and some were more myth than science and should have been recognized as such even in Ramazzini's time. Because of his prestige these fanciful notions must have received wide acceptance and because his book was so admired, **Ramazzini's** influence may have stifled progress in his field during a period when great advances were being made in other branches of medicine. Nevertheless, his cautions to protect workers and his admonition that any doctor called on to treat patients of the working class ask "What occupation does he follow?" earned him the appellation **"Father of Industrial Medicine"**.

For more than 100 years following **Ramazzini's** work, no significant additions to the literature on occupational medicine were published. In the nineteenth century two physicians, **Charles T. Thackrah** in **England** and **Benjamin W. McCready** in **America**, began the modern literature on the recognition of occupational diseases. **McCready's** book, On the Influence of Trades, Professions, and Occupations in the United States, in the Production of Disease, is generally recognized as the first work on occupational medicine published in the United States. The recognition of a causal link between workplace hazards and disease was a key step in the development of the practice of industrial hygiene. The observations by physicians, from Hippocrates to Ramazzini and extending into the twentieth century, of the relationship between work and disease Vernon E. Rose, Dr PH, CIH, CSP, PE History and Philosophy of Industrial Hygiene of occupational medicine.

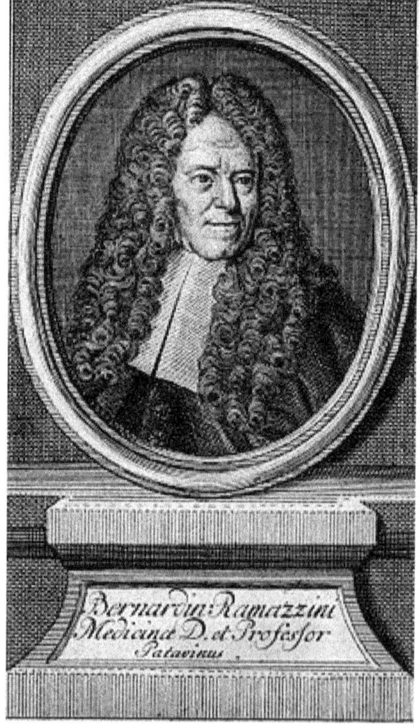

Fig. 1.1 Bernardino Ramazzini

The crystallization of the practice of the profession can be traced to simultaneous developments in Great Britain and the

United States in the late nineteenth and early twentieth centuries. While legislation controlling working conditions was enacted in England beginning in 1802, the early laws were considered totally ineffective, as no proper system of inspection or enforcement was provided.

The **British Factories Act of 1864**, however, required the use of dilution ventilation to reduce air contaminants, while the 1878 version specified the use of exhaust ventilation by fans. The real watershed in industrial medicine and hygiene, however, came in the **British Factories Act of 1901**, which provided for the creation of regulations to control dangerous trades. The development of regulations created the impetus for investigation of workplace hazards and enforcement of control measures. In the **United States in 1905**, the Massachusetts Health Department appointed health inspectors to evaluate dangers of occupations, thus establishing government's role in the nascent field of occupational health. It has been suggested that industrial hygiene did not "emerge as a unique field of endeavour until quantitative measurements of the environment became available.

But in **1910** when **Dr. Alice Hamilton** went, in her own words, "as a pioneer into a new, unexplored field of American medicine, the field of industrial disease Worker exposures to many hazards (e.g., lead and silica) were so excessive and resulting diseases so acute and obvious, the "evaluation" step of industrial hygiene practice required only the sense of sight and an understanding of the concept of cause and effect. This "champion of social responsibility" for worker health and welfare not only presented substantial evidence of a relationship between exposure to toxins and ill health, but also proposed concrete solutions to the problems she encountered.

On an individual basis, Dr. Hamilton's work, which comprised not only the recognition of occupational disease, but the evaluation and control of the causative agents, should be considered as the initial practice of industrial hygiene, at least in the United States. It should be appreciated that many of the early practitioners of industrial hygiene were physicians who, like Alice Hamilton, were interested not only in the diagnosis and treatment of illnesses in industrial workers, but also in hazard control to prevent further cases. These physicians working with engineers and other scientists interested in public health and environmental hazards took the knowledge and insights developed over several millennia from **Hippocrates to Ramazzini, Thackrah and McCready**, and began the process of deliberately changing the work environment with the goal of preventing occupational diseases. What or who then can be designated as representing the origin of the profession? Is there any one person who deserves the title "Founder of Industrial Hygiene"? Certainly, if the name of one individual is sought, that of Alice Hamilton shines like a beacon. But think back to more than 10,000 years ago at the end of the Stone Age, when occupations began to form with the grinding of stone, horn, bone, and ivory tools with sandstone, and with pottery making and linen weaving. Envision a thoughtful worker who suffered from the musculoskeletal problems associated with grinding, made adjustments to his working conditions, and passed the ideas on to co-workers. Recognizing ergonomic problems and solving them would qualify him as an early industrial hygiene practitioner. If that scenario can be imagined, perhaps it is also conceivable that tens of thousands of years ago there was a huntress who recognized the signs and symptoms of anthrax in the bison her group had killed and who made the connection between earlier kills of diseased animals and sickness in members of her tribe. If she then warned her companions of the hazard involved and sought to avoid diseased animals, would she not qualify as one of the founders of the industrial hygiene profession?

If the basic philosophy of the profession is understood, protection of the health and well-being of workers and the public through anticipation, recognition, evaluation, and control of hazards arising in or from the workplace, then the rich tapestry that chronicles the history of industrial hygiene can be imagined. It began when one person recognized a work hazard and took steps not only for self protection, but also for protection of fellow workers. This is the origin and essence of the profession of industrial hygiene.

Historical Events in Industrial Hygiene

1,000,000 BC - Australopithecus used stones as tools and weapons. Flint snappers suffered cuts and eye injuries; bison hunters contracted anthrax.

10,000 BC - Neolithic man began food producing economy and the urban revolution in Mesopotamia. At end of Stone Age, grinding of stone, horn, bone, and ivory tools with sandstone; pottery making, linen weaving. Beginning of the history of occupations.

5000 BC - Copper and Bronze Age - metal workers released from food production. Metallurgy- the first specialized craft.

370 BC - **Hippocrates** dealt with the health of citizens, not workers, but did identify lead poisoning in miners and metallurgists. 50 AD Plinius Secundus (Pliny the Elder) identified use of animal bladders intended to prevent inhalation of dust and lead fume.

200 AD - **Galen** visited a copper mine, but his discussions on public health did not include workers' disease.

Middle Ages No documented contributions to the study of occupational diseases.

1473- **Ellenborg** recognized that the vapours of some metals were dangerous and described the symptoms of industrial poisoning from lead and mercury with suggested preventive measures.

1500 - **In De Re Metallica** (1556), Georgius Agricola described every facet of mining, smelting, and refining, noting prevalent diseases and accidents, and means of prevention including the need for ventilation. Paracelsus (1567) described respiratory diseases among miners with an excellent description of mercury poisoning. Remembered as the father of toxicology. "All substances are poisons . . . the right dose differentiates a poison and a remedy."

1665 - Workday for mercury miners at Idria shortened.

1700 - **Bernardino Ramazzini**, "Father of occupational medicine," published De MorbisArtificumDiatriba, (Diseases of Workers) and examined occupational diseases and "cautions." He introduced the question, "Of what trade are you?"

1775 - **Percival Pott** described occupational cancer among English chimney sweeps, identifying soot and the lack of hygiene measures as a cause of scrotal cancer. The result was the Chimney-Sweeps Act of 1788.

1830 - **Charles Thackrah** authored the first book on occupational diseases to be published in England. His views on disease and prevention helped stimulate factory and health legislation. Medical inspection and compensation were established in 1897.

1900s - **Dr. Alice Hamilton** investigated many dangerous occupations and had tremendous influence on early regulation of occupational hazards in the United States. In 1919 she became the first woman faculty member at Harvard University and wrote exploring the Dangerous Trad.

1902–1911 - Federal and then state (Washington) legislation covering workers' compensation. By 1948 all states covered occupational diseases. First survey in the United States of the extent of occupational disease conducted by the Illinois Occupational Disease Commission. Massachusetts appointed health inspectors to evaluate dangers of occupations.

1910 - First national conference on industrial diseases in the United States.

1912 - **U.S. Congress** levied prohibitive tax on the use of white phosphorus in making matches.

1913 - **National Safety Council** organized. New York and Ohio established first state industrial hygiene agencies.

1914 - **USPHS** organized a Division of Industrial Hygiene and Sanitation. American Public Health Association organized section on industrial hygiene.

1916 - **American Association of Industrial Physicians** and Surgeons formed. American Medical Association held first symposium on industrial hygiene and medicine. 1922 Harvard established industrial hygiene degree program.

1928–1932 - Bureau of Mines conducted toxicological research on solvents, vapours, and gases.

1936 - Walsh-Healy Act required companies supplying goods to government to maintain safe and healthful workplaces.

1938 - National (later American) Conference of Governmental Industrial Hygienists formed.

1939 - American Industrial Hygiene Association organized. American Standards Association and ACGIH prepared first list (maximum allowable concentrations) of standards for chemical exposures in industry.

1941–1945 - Expanded industrial hygiene programs in states. 1941 Bureau of Mines authorized to inspect mines.

1952 - Prof M.N.Rao was the first Indian from Andhra Pradesh who was deputed to International Labour Organisation (ILO) convention to present the Occupational Health status in India.

1960 - American Board of Industrial Hygiene organized by AIHA and ACGIH.

1966 - Metal and Non-metallic Mine Safety Act.

1968 - Professional Code of Ethics drafted by AAIH. Code adopted by all four industrial hygiene associations by 1981.

1969 - Coal Mine Health and Safety Act. 1970 Occupational Safety and Health Act.

1977 - Federal Mine Safety and Health Act. 1992–present Efforts to significantly amend OSH Act. 1995 Revised Professional Code of Ethics adopted by all four industrial hygiene associations.

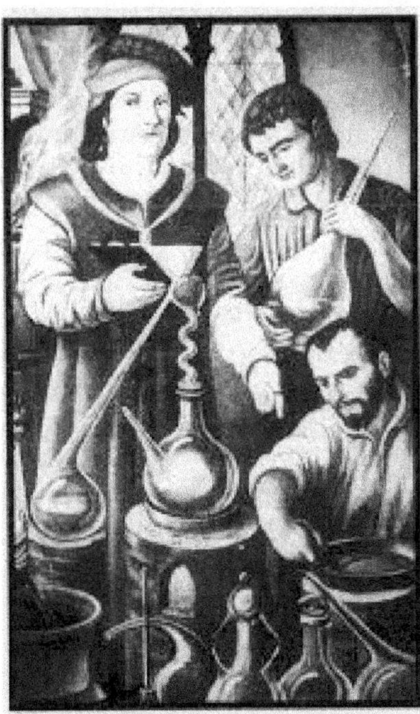

Fig. 1.2 A Portrait of Paracelsus (1567) Who is Remembered as the Father of Toxicology

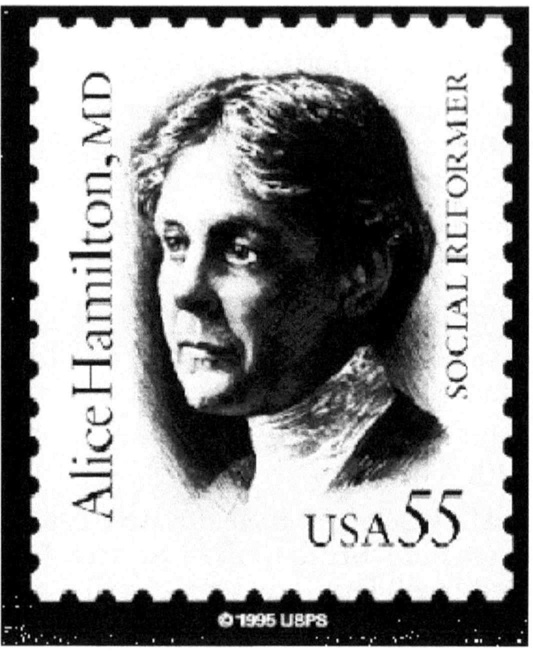

Fig. 1.3 Dr. Alice Hamilton

Science of industrial hygiene flourished in many countries, the United States provided the fertile ground for the development of the profession as it exists today. As the industrial revolution, propelled by the Civil War, progressed in the nineteenth century, individuals began to observe serious health and safety problems (recognition). They also considered the effects on workers (evaluation) and made changes in the work environment (control) to lessen the effects observed. Although these efforts may have resulted in improved worker health and safety, their application was not recognized as the practice of industrial hygiene until the early 1900s. In addition to a chronological listing, these activities also illustrate the concepts of the profession— i.e., recognition, evaluation, and control— which may help to better describe today's practice of industrial hygiene.

1.2 Definitions

Health: Health may be defined as

1. **The state of being free from illness or injury**
2. **A person's mental or physical condition**

3. As defined by World Health Organization (WHO), it is a **"State of complete physical, mental, and social well-being, and not merely the absence of disease or infirmity"**
4. **"The ability to adapt and self-manage"** in the face of social, physical, and emotional challenges
5. **Absence of disease**
6. **The condition of being sound in body, mind or sprit especially freedom from physical disease or pain**

1.2.1 Health

1.2.1.1 The Determinants of Health

Introduction: Many factors combine together to affect the health of individuals and communities. Whether people are healthy or not, is determined by their circumstances and environment. To a large extent, factors such as where we live, the state of our environment, genetics, our income and education level, and our relationships with friends and family all have considerable impacts on health, whereas the more commonly considered factors such as access and use of health care services often have less of an impact.

The determinants of health include:

- **The social and economic environment**
- **The physical environment**
- **The person's individual characteristics and behaviours**

The contexts of people's lives determine their health, and so blaming individuals for having poor health or crediting them for good health is inappropriate. Individuals are unlikely to be able to directly control many of the determinants of health. These determinants or things that make people healthy or not include the above factors, and many others

- ***Income and social status*** - higher income and social status are linked to better health. The greater the gap between the richest and poorest people, the greater the differences in health
- ***Education*** – low education levels are linked with poor health, more stress and lower self-confidence

- ***Physical environment*** – safe water and clean air, healthy workplaces, safe houses, communities and roads all contribute to good health. Employment and working conditions – people in employment are healthier, particularly those who have more control over their working conditions
- ***Social support networks*** – greater support from families, friends and communities is linked to better health. Culture - customs and traditions, and the beliefs of the family and community all affect health
- ***Genetics*** - inheritance plays a part in determining lifespan, healthiness and the likelihood of developing certain illnesses. Personal behaviour and coping skills – balanced eating, keeping active, smoking, drinking, and how we deal with life's stresses and challenges all affect health
- ***Health services*** - access and use of services that prevent and treat disease influences health
- ***Gender*** - Men and women suffer from different types of diseases at different ages

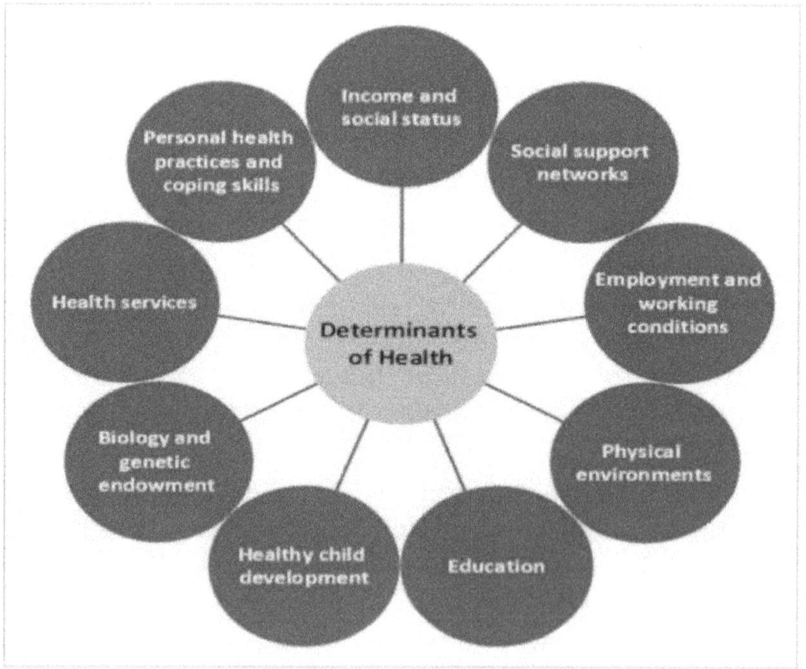

Fig. 1.4 The determinants of health

1.2.1.2 The spectrum of health and illness

To describe health as the absence of disease is inadequate and unsatisfying. We have defined diseases for the last four hundred years or so according to the presence of certain lesions, or the presence of "abnormal" readings measured by instruments of investigation. Illness is a related, but different, term from disease. It is used mainly to refer to the experience of being unwell, incorporating our concept of disease, but actually describing the subjective experience of a person. Only a person can tell you they feel nauseated, or that they have pain. Instruments won't reveal those phenomena.

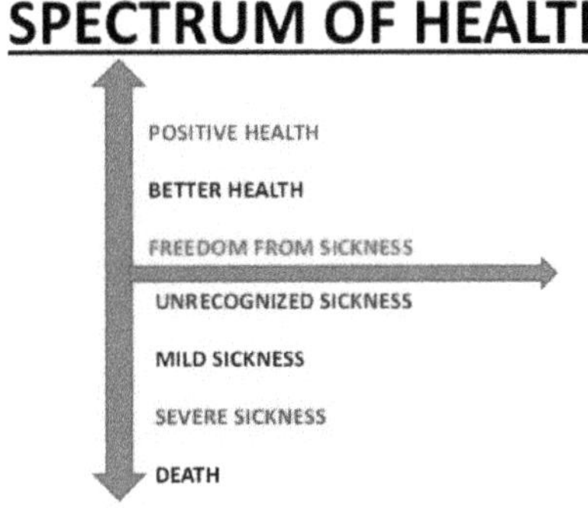

Fig. 1.5 Spectrum of health and illness

1.2.1.3 Factors Effecting Health

1. Social and economic factors
2. Environmental factors (Health)
3. Personal factors
4. Hereditary factors

1. Social and Economic Factors: It depends upon

- Income
- Employment and working conditions
- Food security
- Environment and housing
- Early childhood development
- Education and literacy

2. **Environmental factors (Health):** Environmental health risks are factors outside of the body that can affect a person's wellbeing and influence their behaviour. Examples include the quality of a person's air, food and water supply or their exposure to hazardous materials. Preventing or reducing the risk of illness, injury or disease in the community is essential to good environmental health.

   Examples of environmental health risks

   Environmental health covers many different factors in a person's surroundings. These can include:

   - ***Air pollution*** – for example, smog, wood smoke and mould.
   - ***Water quality*** – for example, grey water, tank water, fluoridation and drought.
   - ***Food quality*** – for example, contamination and nutrition.
   - ***Chemicals*** – for example, pesticides, farm chemicals, arsenic and CCA treated timber.
   - ***Metals*** – for example, exposure to lead, mercury and cadmium.
   - Diseases from animals and insects (vector borne) – for example, dengue fever, hendra virus, lyssavirus, Ross River fever and malaria.
   - Infectious diseases – for example, viral infections like swine flu.

3. **Personal factors:** Personal factors are those which relate to a particular individual and can have an effect on how they act and behave. This obviously has repercussions for overall health and safety as factors such as their attitude, motivation and ability to do the task will all influence the way they work and how. Whilst some personal factors may be ingrained into the person's character and be extremely difficult or even impossible to change, there will be others which can be influenced.

4. **Hereditary Factors:** You might already have a general understanding about heredity that – it is carried from parents to their children and will affect the health and physical characteristics of children. But do you want to know more about what heredity is and how it affects the

health and other physical and mental characteristics? Then we answer in detail to your questions.

We know that genes play an important role in determining our physical characteristics. But to know how genes work, let's get into some biology facts. Cells in human body contain a substance called deoxyribonucleic acid (DNA). DNA is wrapped together to form structures called chromosomes.

1.2.2 Hygiene

Industrial hygiene has been defined as "that science and art devoted to the anticipation, recognition, evolution, and control of those environmental factors or stresses arising in or from the workplace, which may cause sickness, impaired health and well-being, or significant discomfort among workers or among citizens of the community".

1.2.3 Hazard

A hazard is a situation that poses a level of threat to life, health, property, or environment. Most hazards are dormant or potential, with only a theoretical risk of harm; however, once a hazard becomes "active", it can create an emergency situation. A hazardous situation that has come to pass is called an incident. Hazard and possibility interact together to create risk.

Classification of Hazard

Classification of hazard

1. Physical hazard
2. Chemical hazard
3. Biological hazard
4. Ergonomic hazard
5. Psychological hazard

1. ***Physical hazard:*** A physical hazard is a type of occupational hazard that involves environmental hazards that can cause harm with or without contact. Physical hazards include ergonomic hazards, radiation, heat and cold stress, vibration hazards, and noise hazards.

Engineering control are often used to mitigate physical hazards.

Physical hazards are a common source of injuries in many industries. They are perhaps unavoidable in certain industries, such as construction and mining, but over time people have developed safety methods and procedures to manage the risks of physical danger in the workplace. These include excessive levels of ionizing and no ionizing electromagnetic radiation, noise, vibration, illumination, and temperature

In occupations where there is exposure to ionizing radiation, time, distance, and shielding are important tools in ensuring worker safety. Danger from radiation increases with the amount of time one is exposed to it; hence, the shorter the time of exposure the smaller the radiation danger.

Distance also is a valuable tool in controlling exposure to both ionizing and non-ionizing radiation. Radiation levels from some sources can be estimated by comparing the squares of the distances between the worker and the source. For example, at a reference point of 10 feet from a source, the radiation is 1/100 of the intensity at 1 foot from the source.

Shielding also is a way to protect against radiation. The greater the protective mass between a radioactive source and the worker, the lower the radiation exposure.

No ionizing radiation also is dealt with by shielding workers from the source. Sometimes limiting exposure times to no ionizing radiation or increasing the distance is not effective. Laser radiation, for example, cannot be controlled effectively by imposing time limits. An exposure can be hazardous that is faster than the blinking of an eye. Increasing the distance from a laser source may require miles before the energy level reaches a point where the exposure would not be harmful.

Noise, another significant physical hazard, can be controlled by various measures. Noise can be reduced by installing equipment and systems that have been engineered, designed, and built to operate quietly; by enclosing or shielding noisy equipment; by making certain that equipment is in good repair and properly maintained with all worn or unbalanced parts replaced; by mounting noisy equipment on special mounts to reduce vibration; and by installing silencers, mufflers, or baffles.

Substituting quiet work methods for noisy ones is another significant way to reduce noise, for example, welding parts rather than riveting them. Also, treating floors, ceilings, and walls with acoustical material can reduce reflected or reverberant noise. In addition, erecting sound barriers at adjacent work stations around noisy operations will reduce worker exposure to noise generated at adjacent work stations.

It is also possible to reduce noise exposure by increasing the distance between the source and the receiver, by isolating workers in acoustical booths, limiting workers' exposure time to noise, and by providing hearing protection. OSHA requires that workers in noisy surroundings be periodically tested as a precaution against hearing loss.

Another physical hazard, radiant heat exposure in factories such as steel mills, can be controlled by installing reflective shields and by providing protective clothing.

2. ***Chemical hazard:*** Most people automatically associate chemicals with scientists in laboratories, but chemicals are also found in many of the products we use at work and at home. While they have a variety of beneficial uses, chemicals can also be extremely harmful if they are misused.

   Here are some examples of commonly used household products that can damage your health or cause a fire or explosion if used incorrectly:

   - cleaning products such as toilet cleaners, disinfectants, mildew remover and chlorine bleach
   - art supplies, such as paint thinner and pottery glazes
   - garage supplies, such as parts degreasers and cleaning solvents
   - office materials, such as photocopier toner

   Harmful chemical compounds in the form of solids, liquids, gases, mists, dusts, fumes, and vapors exert toxic effects by inhalation (breathing), absorption (through direct contact with the skin), or ingestion (eating or drinking). Airborne chemical hazards exist as concentrations of mists, vapors, gases, fumes, or solids. Some are toxic through inhalation and some of them irritate the skin on contact; some can be toxic by absorption through the skin or through ingestion, and some are corrosive to living tissue.

The degree of worker risk from exposure to any given substance depends on the nature and potency of the toxic effects and the magnitude and duration of exposure.

Information on the risk to workers from chemical hazards can be obtained from the Material Safety Data Sheet (MSDS) that OSHA'S Hazard Communication Standard requires be supplied by the manufacturer or importer to the purchaser of all hazardous materials. The MSDS is a summary of the important health, safety, and toxicological information on the chemical or the mixture's ingredients. Other provisions of the Hazard Communication Standard require that all containers of hazardous substances in the workplace have appropriate warning and identification.

3. ***Biological hazard:*** These include bacteria, viruses, fungi, and other living organisms that can cause acute and chronic infections by entering the body either directly or through breaks in the skin. Occupations that deal with plants or animals or their products or with food and food processing may expose workers to biological hazards. Laboratory and medical personnel also can be exposed to biological hazards. Any occupations that result in contact with bodily fluids pose a risk to workers from biological hazards.

   Sources of biological hazards may include bacteria, viruses, insects, plants, birds, animals, and humans. These sources can cause a variety of health effects ranging from skin irritation and allergies to infections (e.g., tuberculosis, AIDS), cancer and so on. Sources of biological hazards may include bacteria, viruses, insects, plants, birds, animals, and humans. These sources can cause a variety of health effects ranging from skin irritation and allergies to infections (e.g., tuberculosis, AIDS), cancer and so on.

   In occupations where animals are involved, biological hazards are dealt with by preventing and controlling diseases in the animal population as well as proper care and handling of infected animals. Also, effective personal hygiene, hands and forearms, helps keep worker risks to a minimum.

In occupations where there is potential exposure to biological hazards, workers should practice proper personal hygiene, particularly hand washing. Hospitals should provide proper ventilation, proper personal protective equipment such as gloves and respirators, adequate infectious waste disposal systems, and appropriate controls including isolation in instances of particularly contagious diseases such as tuberculosis.

4. ***Ergonomic hazard:*** An ergonomic hazard is a physical factor within the environment that harms the musculoskeletal system. Ergonomic hazards include themes such as monotonous repetitive movements, manual handling, workplace/job/task design, uncomfortable workstation height and poor body positioning.

   The science of ergonomics studies and evaluates a full range of tasks including, but not limited to, lifting, holding, pushing, walking, and reaching. Many ergonomic problems result from technological changes such as increased assembly line speeds, adding specialized tasks, and increased repetition; some problems arise from poorly designed job tasks. Any of those conditions can cause ergonomic hazards such as excessive vibration and noise, eye strain, repetitive motion, and heavy lifting problems. Improperly designed tools or work areas also can be ergonomic hazards. Repetitive motions or repeated shocks over prolonged periods of time as in jobs involving sorting, assembling, and data entry can often cause irritation and inflammation of the tendon sheath of the hands and arms, a condition known as carpal tunnel syndrome.

   Ergonomic hazards are avoided primarily by the effective design of a job or jobsite and better designed tools or equipment that meet workers' needs in terms of physical environment and job tasks. Through thorough worksite analyses, employers can set up procedures to correct or control ergonomic hazards by using the appropriate engineering controls (e.g., designing or re-designing work stations, lighting, tools, and equipment); teaching correct work practices (e.g., proper lifting methods); employing proper administrative controls (e.g., shifting workers among several different tasks, reducing production demand, and increasing rest breaks); and, if necessary, providing and mandating personal protective equipment. Evaluating working conditions from an ergonomics standpoint involves looking at the total physiological and psychological demands of the job on the worker. Overall, industrial hygienists point out that the benefits of a well-designed, ergonomic work environment can include increased efficiency, fewer accidents, lower operating costs and more effective use of personnel.

In sum, industrial hygiene encompasses a broad spectrum of the working environment. Early in its history OSHA recognized industrial hygiene as an integral part of a healthful work setting. OSHA places a high priority on using industrial hygiene concepts in its health standards and as a tool for effective enforcement of job safety and health regulations. By recognizing and applying the principles of industrial hygiene to the work environment, America's workplaces will become more healthful and safer.

5. ***Psychological hazard*:** Psychosocial hazards include but aren't limited to stress, violence and other workplace stressors. Work is generally beneficial to mental health and personal wellbeing. It provides people with structure and purpose and a sense of identity. It also provides opportunities for people to develop and use their skills, to form social relationships, and to increase their feelings of self-worth.

   There are circumstances, however, in which work can have adverse consequences for health and wellbeing. Risks to psychological health at work may arise from organizational or personal factors, with the major factors being poor design of work and jobs, poor communication and interpersonal relationships, bullying, occupational violence and fatigue. Risks to psychological health due to work should be viewed in the same way as other health and safety risks and a commitment to prevention of work-related stress should be included in an organization's health and safety policies.

   A psychological hazard is any hazard that affects the mental well-being or mental health of the worker and may have physical effects by overwhelming the individual coping mechanisms and impacting the workers ability to work in a healthy and safe manner. Although these issues have been around for many years, psychosocial hazards are only now being recognized as potential workplace hazards. The hazards generally are not from physical things that you can see (like a saw blade) or smell (like paint). Rather, many of these hazards come about as a result of interactions with others. In some cases, the hazard is brought into the workplace from the home. There are often no obvious outward signs of the effects of exposure and the methods to control these hazards are somewhat different than methods used to control other traditional workplace hazards.

The types of issues or concerns included in this category are:

- Fatigue and hours of work
- Technological changes
- Stress and critical incident stress
- Bullying including cyber bulling/harassment
- Workplace violence and abuse

1.2.4 Occupational Disease

An occupational disease is any chronic ailment that occurs as a result of work or occupational activity. It occurs as a result of exposure to physical, chemical, biological and psychological factor in the work place.

- Occupational diseases have a long latent period
- Most occupational diseases cannot be treated be prevented
- All occupational diseases can

Some of the well-known Occupational disease are as follows

- Silicosis
- Asbestosis
- Bagassosis
- Byssinosis
- Dermatitis
- Anthrax

- Pneumoconiose
- Lead poisoning
- Occupational cancer

1.3 Control Measure

1. Elimination
2. Substitution
3. Engineering Controls
4. Administrative Controls
5. Personnel Protective Equipment (PPE)

To control the hazards there are four principles in general. Elimination of the best option, if elimination is not possible then substitution should be Engineering control is applied to control hazards by engineering modifications in the process. The last principle advocates the administrative control by making some administrative mechanism in the workplace to keep away hazards from human and workplace.

The application of all four control measures with the use of personal protective equipment (PPEs) reduces the hazards significantly in workplace and outside of the unit.

1.3.1 Elimination

The most effective control measure is to control hazards at the source by eliminating the hazard. Eliminate hazards at the "development stage" it is important to consider health and safety aspects when work processes are still in the planning stages. For example, when purchasing machines, safety should be the first concern, not cost. Machines should conform to national safety standards — they should be designed with the correct guard on them to eliminate the danger of a worker getting caught in the machine while using it. Machines that are not produced with the proper guards on them may cost less to purchase, but cost more in terms of accidents, loss of production, compensation, etc. Unfortunately, many used machines that do not meet safety standards are exported to developing countries, causing workers to pay the price with accidents, hearing loss from noise, etc.

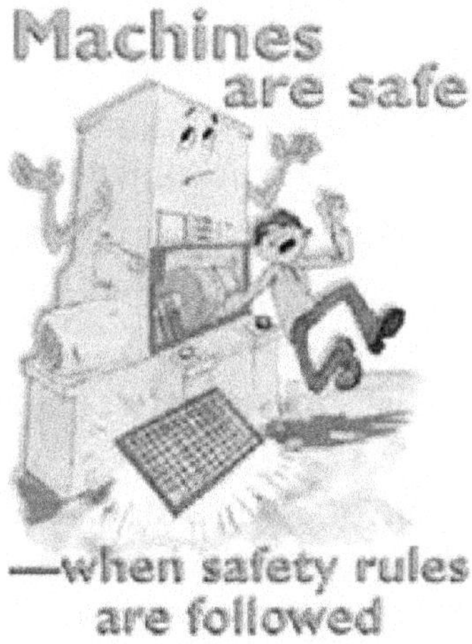

The above figure is one example for accident when machine guard is eliminated, in other words, a hazard of an accident could be eliminated by providing the machine guard.

Any avoidable exposure to dangerous substances should be eliminated.

Some hints on where to look

- Regarding hazards caused by the process
- Open processes, e.g. painting big surfaces, Mixing/ compounding in open containers/vessels
- Processes generating dusts, vapours or fumes or dispersing liquids in the air e.g. welding, spraying paint
- Related to the substance
- If you cannot change the work process, try to eliminate or avoid the exposure for substances that
- Increase fire and explosion risks;
- Leads to high exposure of workers
- Results in exposure to many workers
- Are volatile, e.g., organic solvents
- Are dispersed in the air (aerosols, dust)
- Cause acute health risks, e.g., poisons, corrosives and irritants

- Cause chronic health risks, such as allergens, substances toxic for reproduction and others
- Are covered by specific national regulations imposing restrictions of use in the workplace
- Have already caused problems in your enterprise (health problems, accidents orother incidents);
- Cause occupational diseases
- Make regular health monitoring (medical examination of workers) necessary
- Can be absorbed through the skin or substances for which the use of personal protective equipment impairing workers (e.g. inhalation protection) is necessary

1.3.2 Substitution

Substitution of currently-used materials with less hazardous materials is one of the most effective ways of eliminating or reducing exposure to materials that are toxic or pose other hazards. A hazard is the source of danger or injury. A hazard includes any chemical or material that has the ability or a property that can cause an adverse health effect or harm to a person under certain conditions. Risk, on the other hand, is the probability or chance that exposure to a chemical hazard will actually cause harm to a person or cause an adverse effect.

Other occupational hygiene methods for controlling employee exposure to chemicals include isolation, enclosure, local exhaust ventilation, process or equipment modification, good housekeeping, administrative controls and personal protective equipment. All these methods reduce or eliminate the risk of injury or harm by interrupting the path of exposure between the hazardous material and the worker. Substitution removes the hazard at the source.

Why should the substitute material be chosen very carefully?

Extreme care must be taken to ensure that one hazard is not being exchanged for another, especially one that could even be a more serious hazard. Before deciding to replace a chemical, one must know the risks of the chemical to the employees, the environment, and the risks for damage to equipment and facilities. If the risks are serious, then alternatives should be considered and their risks must also be understood.

The selection of a substitute can be a very complex process. In large organizations the selection process may involve a committee with representatives from engineering, purchasing, industrial hygiene, safety, maintenance, research and development, environmental control, waste management, shipping and the supervisors and workers who directly work with the material. In smaller organizations, one person may carry out many of these functions.

Substitution Process

General considerations

Substitution may be an isolated event in a company or it may be part of a more systematic approach or policy at company/sector or local/regional level.

It should be integrated in the general policies and plans of companies, making good use of existing knowledge within the companies and of the relations with external stakeholders (partners, authorities, shareholders, supply chain, clients).

Making substitution part of the preventive culture of the company helps to identify problems earlier - spotting opportunities, acting in a coherent way and gaining broader support.

Multidisciplinary teams are generally needed, depending on the nature and complexity of the substitution. Such teams should include preventive services and occupational physicians, technical personnel, and workers representatives.

Workers have to be informed, encouraged and involved in identifying possible substitutions and discussing the appropriateness of their implementation, as well as when putting them into practice. The fact that substitution is a change (sometimes an innovation) may be stimulating in some cases, but in others it will challenge companies' and workers´ capacities to adapt, to change mindsets, and to control things while under development. Information exchange along the supply chain or at sector level can promote substitution initiatives and share practical experience.

The right timing for substitution is influenced by the availability and the costs of substitution. Big companies can afford to make a competitive advantage of putting on the market or using a new and safer alternative, even while prices are still high. Small companies might need to wait for prices to go down.

A critical issue is the current state of knowledge on the long-term effects of substances. In some notorious cases, like asbestos, chemicals were proven unsafe after many years of intensive use. Such cases make it hard to decide on implementing alternatives, especially when they are not supported by long-term epidemiological studies. Constant improvement of laboratory tests and modeling methods are expected to provide more reliable data and in shorter time. A precautionary approach is recommended, and substitution by unknown substances should be avoided until clarification is forthcoming, in particular if the current risk is low and may not justify such a step.

A risk assessment for the alternative should determine if risk is reduced, and what protective measures are required. An alternative will rarely be the safest for all hazard endpoints. Decision on what alternative to adopt should consider which hazard is more likely to generate high risks levels, and which one the company is better able to control. As well as chemical risks, other risks should also be considered that could impact negatively on health and safety (e.g. risk of fire and explosion risks). The impact on the main working processes and on auxiliary activities like maintenance should be considered, as well as the consequences of possible accidents. Working procedures, protective and preventive measures already in place may need to be amended or supplemented. Companies could develop purchasing procedures to select for safer chemicals and products as they become available.

The principle of substitution to avoid chemicals of high concern can also be applied to the design of new products or processes, which is a preferable preventive approach.

Substitution Steps

The following steps are general and indicative, and can be adjusted, if appropriate, to bring about the desired result:

- ***Organising a working group:*** Insure appropriate representation of workers and employers, and integrate all required expertise. Include those directly involved in using/producing the substance (technicians, workers). Make a work plan with well-defined roles for all stages. Take measures to ensure an efficient information flow between the group, the rest of the company and its stakeholders. Maintain a collaborative, open–minded atmosphere.
- ***Defining the problem:*** List the substances to be substituted. Be clear on why you make these choices. Priorities substitutions according to legal provisions, company policy and stakeholder perspective. Define the function that a substance has and how it is integrated in the rest of the process/product. List the required conditions for this function to perform adequately (temperature, acidity, pressure, chemical compatibility, etc.). An alternative should fit these conditions, or the system/product will need to be changed, to a greater or lesser degree. Define what quality the substance gives to the process or to the final product. If that quality is not actually necessary needed (e.g. some commercial attributes) the substance may be eliminated. Otherwise, an alternative is needed.
- ***Setting substitution criteria:*** Set criteria for selecting possible alternatives. Initially, fewer (pre)screening criteria may be used. This would eliminate at an early stage those alternatives that are not safe enough CMRs and substances of equivalent concern, such as endocrine disruptors, also sensitizers or neurotoxin ants should not be chosen as alternatives. Other criteria may be added to differentiate between alternatives that have passed the screening criteria. Cost, availability on the local market, and other advantages may be considered.
- ***Searching for alternatives:*** Solutions may be found inside the company. Searching other sources is also important. Alternatives already developed and implemented may lower innovation costs and risks. Internet sources, official reports, supplier chain, professional or sectorial associations or authority representatives may provide

useful information. Another approach is to ask the supplier to formulate a safer alternative. Some companies offer support in selecting the right product, or may even be willing to reformulate the initial one (especially for important clients).

- ***Assessing and comparing alternatives:*** Assess all alternatives using the same method or tool to allow for comparison. Select those alternatives that best fit the nature and dimension of the problem and that provide indeed an overall risk reduction.
- ***Experimenting on pilot scale:*** Try substitution on a smaller scale to see if it lives up to expectations in terms of safety, technical and environmental performance. Compare costs against those initially forecast, and estimate if feasible when transposed at full scale.
- ***Implementing, Re-evaluating:*** Plan carefully for full scale implementation. Evaluate the risks (see also: Risk Assessment Tool) and take appropriate measures. Review as necessary the supply chain, training needs, monitoring (see also: Air Monitoring), and other procedures.

The table below provides some examples:

Instead of	Consider
Carbon tetrachloride (causes liver damage, cancer)	1,1,1-trichloroethane, dichloromethane
Benzene (causes cancer)	Toluene, cyclohexane, ketones
Pesticides (causes various effects on body)	"Natural" pesticides such as pyrethrums
Organic solvents (causes various effects on body)	Water-detergent solutions
Leaded glazes, paints, pigments (causes various effects on body)	Versions that do not contain lead
Sandstone grinding wheels (causes severe respiratory illness due to silica)	Synthetic grinding wheels such as aluminium oxide

Remember, however, that you need to make sure the substitute chemical or substance is not causing any harmful effects and to control and monitor exposures to make sure that the replacement chemical or substance is below occupational exposure limits.

Another type of substitution includes using the same chemical but to use it in a different form. For example, a dry, dusty powder may be a significant inhalation hazard but if this material can be purchased and used as pellets or crystals, there may be less dust in the air and therefore less exposure.

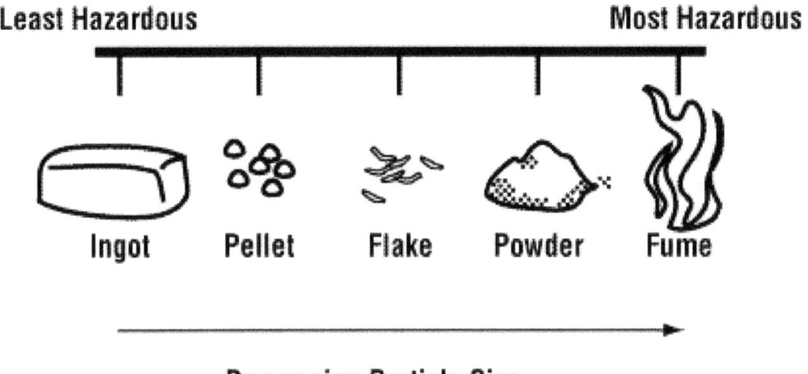

Fig. 1.6 Hazard based on size

When substituting, be very careful that one hazard is not being traded for another. Before deciding to replace a chemical/substance with another, consider all the implications and potential risks of the new material.

Elimination or substitution can lead to

- Improved immediate and long-term health of the workers exposed to the dangerous substance;
- Reduced pollution of the environment;
- Reduced costs to the enterprise by:
- Lowering sickness absence,
- Spending less on control measures,
- Reduced cost in compliance with environmental legislation,
- Saving money on fire and explosion protection,
- Lower consumption of a product,
- Using cheaper materials,
- More efficient work processes

The variety of substitutions and their context are presented in the examples below.

Construction sector - substitution by non chemical alternative - personal initiative in an SME:

A worker in a SME proposed the use of an electric, infrared (IR) heater to soften old paint, instead of the usual chemical procedure for stripping, based on dichloromethane. Initially, the proposal had nothing to do with occupational safety or environmental protection. The IR stripper was easier to transport, store and use than the chemicals. The substitution was well received by co-workers, who soon also noticed the OSH advantages. Moreover, unlike torch stripers, the IR device does not develop temperatures that volatilize hazardous components such as lead; nor does it create dusts, like mechanical methods (e.g. blasting). When the SME proposed it in its next subcontract offer as a "green solution", it made a good impression on the contractor and the beneficiary.

Health care sector - substitution by product changes (packaging) and organizational measures - part of a broader risk reduction plan.

As part of the process to eliminate mercury in health care units, a hospital decided to use thimerosal free vaccines. Thimerosal (or thiomersal) is a mercury-containing preservative that stabilizes vaccines. Using preservative free vaccines meant changing the supplying procedure: single vials instead of multiple vial vaccines were used, and the storing time was shortened. The hospital reduced chemicals risks and hazardous wastes waste, and patients that rejected vaccines containing mercury were reassured.

Chemical industry - substitution by chemical - large company.

One of the biggest manufacturers of chemicals synthesized 1,2-Cyclohexane dicarboxylic acid diisononyl ester (DINCH) as an alternative to phthalate plasticisers such as bis(2-ethylhexyl)phthalate (DEHP) which is classified as reprotoxicant and endocrine disruptor in the EU and as possibly carcinogenic to humans by the International Agency for Research on Cancer. Released in 2002, it has been used successfully in sensitive applications such as medical devices, children's products, and food. Today it is one of the most used alternatives to phthalate plasticisers.

Other examples are:

- Electric motors instead of diesel or petrol engines to eliminate hazardous exhaust fumes;
- "Dust-free" cutting or grinding equipment;
- Dip or brush instead of spray painting;
- Covered containers to carry materials which produce air contaminants.
- Use a vacuum cleaning when cleaning up toxic dust. Never sweep toxic dust-sweeping puts the dangerous dust back into the air where you can breathe it.

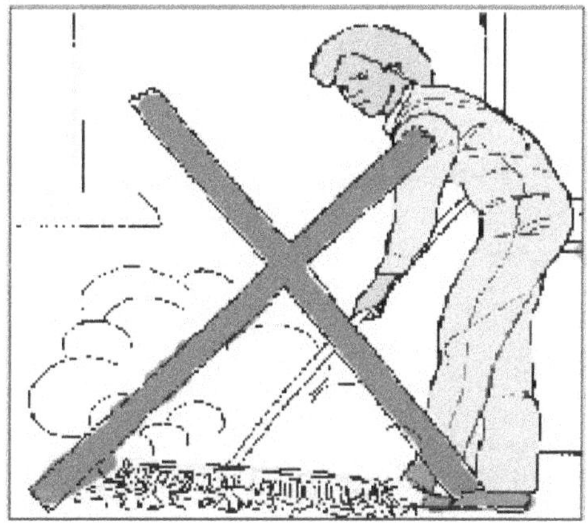

- Demolition of structure using mechanical sheers; combined with the safe work practice of spraying water will significantly reduce worker exposure to harmful dust.

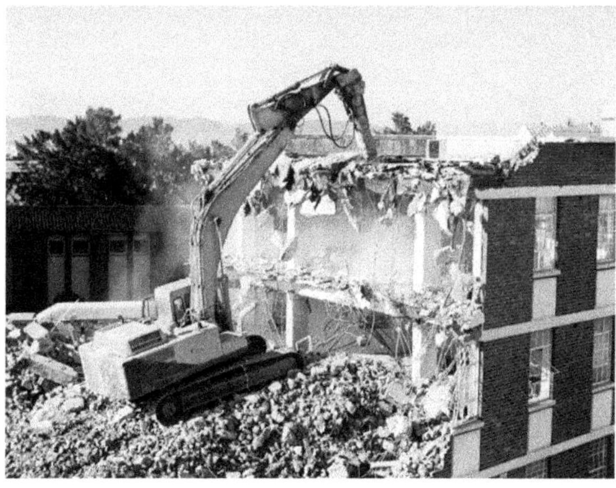

1.3.3 Change in the Process

Hierarchy of Controls

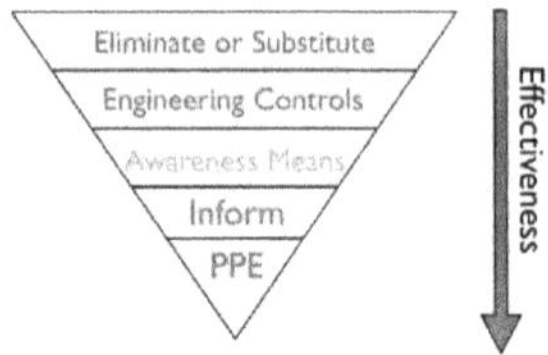

Change the Process

If there are no reliable substitutes for dangerous chemicals, then you can consider changing the way the process is carried out. It may be possible to change the process so that it makes the handling of substances safer. Example: using a wet method to control dust; or steam cleaning instead of solvents. Hand operated controls on the production line should be closer so that workers do not have to bend or stretch.

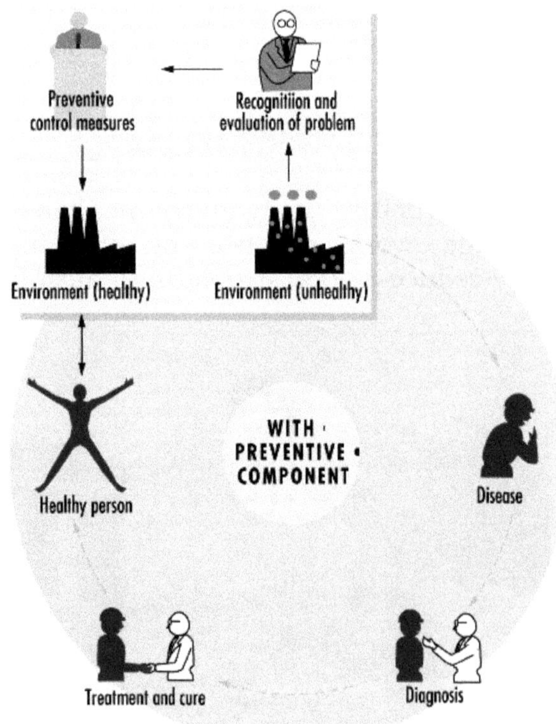

Mechanise the Process

Certain dangerous work can be automated. This will prevent workers from going near the dangerous substance or process.

Example: Instead of manual dipping of metal parts in a degreaser, one can use an automatic parts process.

Measurements for Control

Measurements with the purpose of investigating the presence of agents and the patterns of exposure parameters in the work environment can be extremely useful for the planning and design of control measures and work practices. The objectives of such measurements include:

- Source identification and characterization
- Spotting of critical points in closed systems or enclosures (e.g., leaks)
- Determination of propagation paths in the work environment
- Comparison of different control interventions
- Verification that reparable dust has settled together with the coarse visible dust, when using water sprays
- Checking that contaminated air is not coming from an adjacent area.

Direct-reading instruments are extremely useful for control purposes, particularly those which can be used for continuous sampling and reflect what is happening in real time, thus disclosing exposure situations which might not otherwise be detected and which need to be controlled. Examples of such instruments include: photo-ionization detectors, infrared analysers, aerosol meters and detector tubes. When sampling to obtain a picture of the behaviour of contaminants, from the source throughout the work environment, accuracy and precision are not as critical as they would be for exposure assessment.

Measurements are also needed to assess the efficiency of control measures. In this case, source sampling or area sampling are convenient, alone or in addition to personal sampling, for the assessment of workers' exposure. In order to assure validity, the locations for "before" and "after" sampling (or measurements) and the techniques used should be the same, or equivalent, in sensitivity, accuracy and precision.

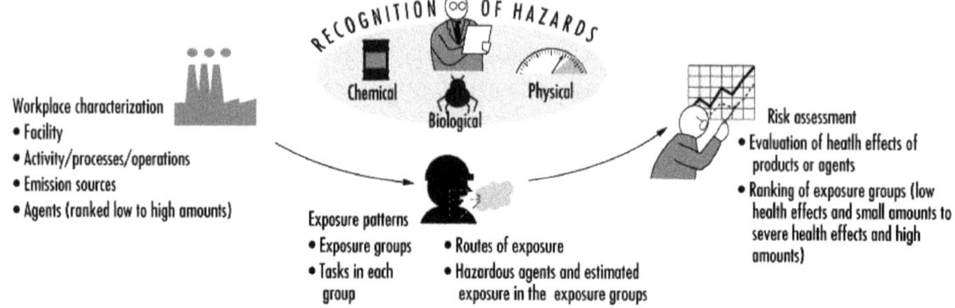

Fig. 1.7 Recognition of Hazards

Occupational Health

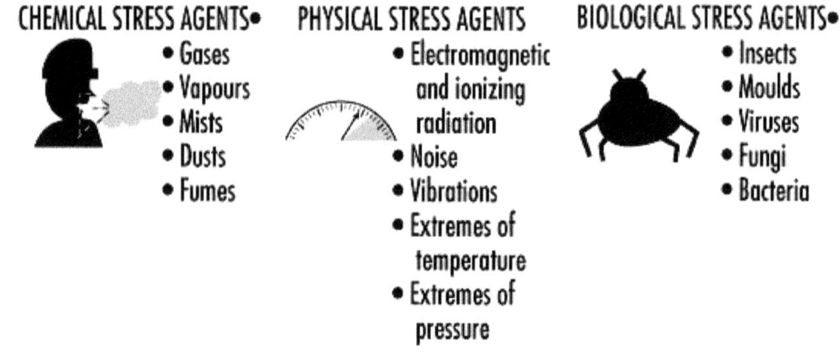

Fig. 1.8 Occupational Health stress agents

These stress removed in industrial and construction areas for better health.

Workplace Assessment Methods

Although there are many aspects to occupational hygiene work the most known and sought after is in determining or estimating potential or actual exposures to hazards. For many chemicals and physical hazards, occupational exposure limits have been derived using toxicological, epidemiological and medical data allowing hygienists to reduce the risks of health effects by implementing the "Hierarchy of Hazard Controls". Several methods can be applied in assessing the workplace or environment for exposure to a known or suspected hazard.

Occupational hygienists do not rely on the accuracy of the equipment or method used but in knowing with certainty and precision the limits of the equipment or method being used and the error or variance given by using that particular equipment or method. Well known methods for performing occupational exposure assessments can be found in "A Strategy for Assessing and Managing Occupational Exposures".

The main steps outlined for assessing and managing occupational exposures:

- Basic Characterization (identify agents, hazards, people potentially exposed and existing exposure controls).
- Exposure Assessment (select occupational exposure limits, hazard bands, relevant toxicological data to determine if exposures are "acceptable", "unacceptable" or "uncertain")
- Exposure Controls (for "unacceptable" or "uncertain" exposures)
- Further Information Gathering (for "uncertain" exposures)
- Hazard Communication (for all exposures)
- Reassessment (as needed) / Management of Change.

Need for Re-Validation

There are many changes that could lead to a need to re-validate a control measure or combination of control measures. Examples include:

System failure

If monitoring or verification identifies failures for which a process deviation cause cannot be identified, re-validation may be needed. Non-compliance with monitoring or verification criteria may indicate a need for a change in the parameters (i.e., the selection and specification of the control measures) on which the design of the food safety control system is based. A system failure may also result from an inadequate hazard analysis and may require re-validation.

Process changes

The introduction in the food safety control system of a new control measure, technology or a piece of equipment that is likely to have a decisive impact on the control of the hazard may necessitate that the system or parts of it be re-validated.

Similarly, changes made in product formulation or the application of current control measures (e.g. time/temperature changes) may result in the need for re-validation of control measures.

New scientific or regulatory information:

- Re-validation may be needed if the hazard associated with a food or ingredient changes as a result of higher concentrations of hazards than originally encountered and accounted for in the design
- A change in response of a hazard to control (e.g. adaptation)
- 10 Decision criteria should take into account the uncertainty and variability associated with the validation methodology and the performance of the control measure or combination of control measure

Isolation

Definition - What does Isolation mean?

Isolation, in the context of databases, specifies when and how the changes implemented in an operation become visible to other parallel operations. Transaction isolation is an important part of any transactional system. It deals with consistency and completeness of data retrieved by queries unreflecting a user data by other user actions. A database acquires locks on data to maintain a high level of isolation.

Enclosed operations

Isolation of the source of exposure can be accomplished through actual physical enclosure, preferably separate rooms or buildings, and closed doors. The direction of airflow must be into the restricted area from the cleaner areas. Therefore, the isolated area must be under negative pressure compared to surrounding areas. This is accomplished by exhausting extra air from the isolated area to the outdoors using fans in either general or local exhaust ventilation.

Exhaust air must be decontaminated before release to the outdoors. There should be no connections between the isolated area and other areas via the ventilation system, ceiling plenums, pipe chase ways, openings in walls, etc.

Regulated areas

As a further precaution, regulated areas can be established around enclosed operations with access only to a limited number of essential employees. Entrances to regulated areas should be posted informing workers that the areas may be entered only by authorized personnel and the special procedures, such as wearing respirators that must be followed in the regulated area. A roster of employees entering and leaving the regulated area should be kept. No smoking, eating, drinking, chewing tobacco or gum, or applying cosmetics is permitted in regulated areas. Air locks with interlocked doors add an extra measure of isolation. Computerized card readers and doors with alarms prevent unauthorized entry.

Isolation by time

The amount of time employees spend in isolated or regulated areas should be minimized. A hazardous operation can sometimes be performed during the second or third shift to reduce the number or workers potentially exposed.

Glove boxes

Glove boxes are usually small units that have two or more ports in which arm-length rubber gloves are mounted. The worker places her hands in these gloves to perform tasks inside the box. Construction materials vary widely, depending on the intended use. Clear plastic is frequently used because it allows visibility of the work area and is easily cleaned. Glove boxes generally operate under negative pressure so that any air leakage is into the box. Exhaust air must be decontaminated. Because these units have low airflow, scrubbing or absorption of exhaust air can be accomplished with little difficulty.

Enclose workers

Workers can be protected by enclosure in a special isolated booth or room from which they can observe and control an operation using chemicals. One disadvantage of this method is the social isolation of the worker. Worker enclosures should be as roomy and comfortable as possible. They should be provided with heating and air conditioning and provided with clean air from an uncontaminated location. They should be under positive pressure to keep out contamination.

Isolate Best practice

- Requirements must be established for conducting these activities in job instructions or method descriptions, for instance.
- It is important that somebody is responsible for process isolation, and that this person approves the start of isolation. This person will also coordinate the sequence of activities if several people are responsible for the isolation job.
- The people doing the job must discuss and understand the underlying philosophy of the isolation plan before starting work. This could be accomplished, for example, by the responsible operations supervisor going through and explaining the plan to the relevant personal.

Execution

- A physical barrier must always be in place to prevent actuator-controlled valves from changing position. The isolation method must be sufficiently secure to provide assurance that for example a loss of power or air will not change the valve position.
- Because of the above, a quality-assured overview with tag number showing how each valve is to be isolated should be available for each individual platform/facility. This overview will form the basis for executing isolations.
- Tagging campaigns. Ensuring that all equipment – not only valves, but also connections and other relevant items – is tagged represents a crucial requirement. Tagging campaigns should accordingly be pursued. This work can possibly be outsourced to contractors.
- Consequences of missing tags. A lack of tagging should generate a requirement for physical checking the plant. This must be done by at least two people.
- Setting specific expertise requirements for those doing the isolation is important. (Similar requirements must apply for those verifying isolations.)

- If isolation and leak testing are conducted in parallel, these, activities must be performed systematically (finishing work on one barrier/component before continuing to the next).
- A system must be in place for labelling the involved, equipment, checking that isolation has been carried out and has not been altered by others. - Labels must be hung on the equipment as the isolation process proceeds. A system must be in place to ensure that the quantity of labels and the number on each 11 accords with the isolation plan. This will help to ensure that no items on the plan are overlooked. Example: a dedicated printer connected to the WP system.
- Locking. Some companies have routines for locking valves so that their position cannot be inadvertently changed by others (see below).
- Isolation should be carried out at a time when sufficient peace and quiet prevails for a thorough job to be done.
- The list of break sections must be updated if breaking of flanges or removal of plugs forms part of the isolation process. This list must be a dynamic document which specifies at any given time which points (both flanges and plugs) have been broken.

Purging

Purging should always be done before work starts on hydrocarbon equipment. That also applies to work on safety valves.

Bledding

- Common specifications should apply for all hoses, so thatusing the "wrong" one will not have significant consequences.
- Requirements must be set for the way the hose ends are to be secured so that they do not dance around in the event of a leak.
- Proposals on best practice for bleeding have been prepared (see below).
- Criteria on what is to be regarded as a safe area for bleeding must be prepared for each facility.
- Requirements must be established for the way verification

Verify Isolations

- Is to be performed
- Verification must always be required, even if the isolation only embraces a few valves
- Measures to ensure that the verifier is conscious of their role are recommended. Efforts must be made to achieve the best possible verification

Approved Isolations

- It is important that the responsible operations supervisor Approve isolations have expertise about the systems involved in the isolation.
- Examples of checkpoints which the responsible operations supervisor must verbally ensure have been performed are provided in an appendix to this document.

Demonstrate Zero Energy

Routines must be in place to demonstrate zero energy for the person who is to do the job. This involves, for example, demonstrating that the system is depressurised by opening and closing a valve, trying to start pumps which have been disconnected and which form part of the isolation, and so forth

Enclosure and Isolation

- These methods aim to keep the chemical "in" and the worker "out" (or vice versa).
- An enclosure keeps a selected hazard "physically" away from the worker. Enclosed equipment, for example, is tightly sealed and it is typically only opened for cleaning or maintenance. Other examples include "glove boxes" (where a chemical is in a ventilated and enclosed space and the employee works with the material by using gloves that are built in), abrasive blasting cabinets, or remote control devices. Care must be taken when the enclosure is opened for maintenance as exposure could occur if adequate precautions are not taken. The enclosure itself must be well maintained to prevent leaks.
- Isolation places the hazardous process "geographically" away from the majority of the workers. Common isolation techniques are to create a contaminant-free booth either around the equipment or around the employee workstations.

Isolation and Enclosure

The principal of isolation is frequently envisioned as being limited to installation of a physical barrier between hazardous operation and the workers. However isolated can be provided without a physical barrier by appropriate use of time and distance.

1.3.4 Reduce Exposure Time

There is a simple relationship between the length of time a person is exposed to a hazardous substance and the dose of substance that they receive: double the time, double the dose; half the time, half the dose. It is therefore sensible to minimize the time period over which people work with hazardous substances, especially where those substances can have an acute effect. Exposure may also be limited by occupational exposure limits.

1.3.5 Enclosure and Segregation

It may be necessary to totally enclose the hazardous substance. The aim here is to isolate the hazard physically so that nobody is exposed to it. This might be done by total enclosure or containment of the hazard. e.g. creating an acoustic enclosure of a noisy machine to reduce the noise reaching those nearby.

Segregation is simply placing the hazard in an inaccessible location. It might be stored in a segregated storage area and used in an area away from other work processes and unauthorized personnel.

1.3.6 Wet Method

Wet method is one of the oldest and effective methods for controlling exposures to dust is the practice of wetting or spraying the operation or dusty area to clean by use of sprinkler system. Such wet methods are common at dusty construction sites, in sand casting operations and at quarrying operations. Sweeping operation in plants can be performed more cleanly and with less dust generation by wetting the area before sweeping. This can also make it easier to collect and prepare the material for proper disposal. It is a very effective method to control employee exposure during asbestos handing, removal, cutting, and cleanup except where the use of wet method are not feasible or will create safety hazards.

Some studies have shown that wet cutting methods can reduce average repairable dust levels by up to 94%. However, if an Employer determines that the use of a wet saw in a particular circumstance is not feasible, and the brick, concrete block or Masonry must be cut dry, and then the employer would be required to explore other engineering control options. Dust collection systems can be used, but they are typically not sufficient to reduce exposures below permissible limits and employees will usually need to be protected with appropriate respirators as well; monitoring the air will confirm exposure.

1.3.7 Local Exhaust Ventilation

Local exhaust ventilation (LEV) is an engineering system frequently used in the workplace to protect employees from hazardous substances. Local exhaust ventilation (LEV) is only one of many engineering control options that may be used to remove and prevent employee exposure to vapor, mist, dust or other airborne contaminants. To have an effective system it is important that it is well designed and installed, used correctly and properly maintained.

Ventilation is a method of control that strategically "adds" and "removes" air in the work environment. Ventilation can remove or dilute an air contaminant if designed properly. Local exhaust ventilation is very adaptable to almost all chemicals and operations. It removes the contaminant at the source so it cannot disperse into the workspace and it generally uses lower exhaust rates than general ventilation (general ventilation usually exchanges air in the entire room).Local exhaust ventilation is an effective means of controlling hazardous exposures but should be used when other methods (such as elimination or substitution) are not possible.
A local exhaust ventilation system consists of these basic parts:

- **Hoods** - A hood that captures the contaminants generated in the air (at the source). Collection point for gathering the contaminated air into the system.
- **Duct** - Ductwork that carries the contaminated air to the air cleaning device, if present or to the fan (away from the

source).To transport the extracted air to the purifying device or the outside atmosphere.

- **Fan** - A fan which draws the air from the hood into the ducts and removes the air from the workspace. The fan must overcome all the losses due to friction, hood entry, and fittings in the system while producing the intended flow rate.
- **Air purifying device** - Air cleaning devices may also be present that can remove contaminants such as dust), gases and vapours from the air stream before it is discharged or exhausted into the environment depending on the material(s) being used in the hood. Such as charcoal filters are often used to remove organic chemical contaminants.

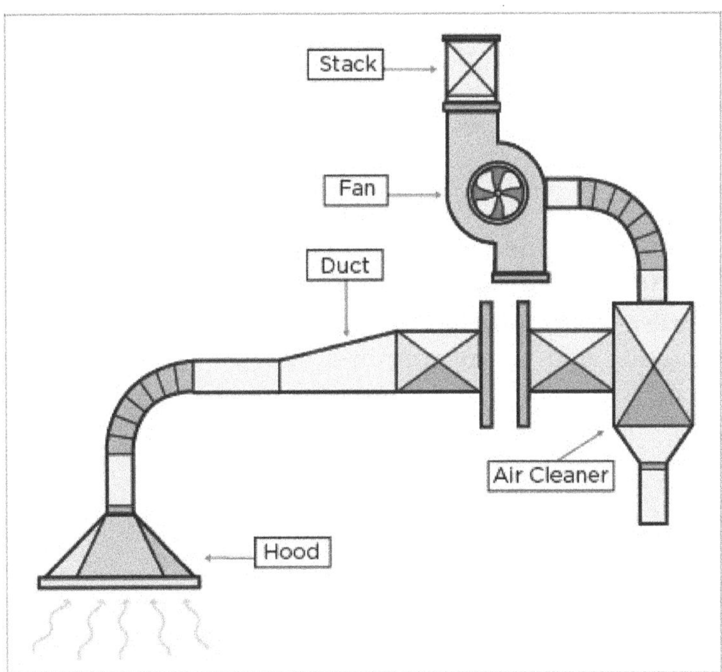

Fig. 1.9 Local Exhaust Ventilation

The design of a ventilation system is very important and must match the particular process and chemical or contaminant in use. Expert guidance should be sought. It is a very effective control measure but only if it is designed, tested, and maintained properly. Because contaminants are exhausted to the outdoors, you should also check with your local environment ministry or municipality for any environmental air regulations or bylaws that may apply in your area.

1.3.8 Dilution Ventilation

Dilution ventilation operates by diluting the contaminant concentration in the general atmosphere to an acceptable level by changing the air efficiently in the workplace over a given period of time. This system is intended to remove gas contaminants (sometimes fumes) and keep the overall concentration of any contaminants to below the occupational exposure limits (OEL).

Dilution ventilation is appropriate where

- The OEL of the harmful substance is high
- The rate of formation of the gas or vapour is slow
- Operators are not in close contact with contamination generation point.
- If a powered system is used, fans must be appropriately sited. If the contaminant is
- **Lighter than air**, it will naturally rise up inside workrooms and can be extracted at a high level.
- **Heavier than air**, it will sink to the floor and low level extraction will be appropriate.

CHAPTER 2

Personal Hygiene

2.1 Importance of Personal Hygiene

Hygiene

Hygiene is received from the Greek word "hygies" (Hygiea-Goddess of Health) Meaning "healthy, sound"

The concept of hygiene dates back to the time when first man has moved into the caves to protect himself from the forces of nature that acts against his survival. The concept of hygiene as an art is as old as the history of mankind although nowadays it has been recognized as a science of its own.

Personal Hygiene

It may be described as the principle of maintaining cleanliness and grooming of the external body. Failure to keep up a standard of hygiene can have many implications. Not only is there an increased risk of getting an infection or illness, but there are many social and psychological aspects that can be affected.

Personal hygiene is a concept that is commonly used in medical and public health practices. It is also widely practiced at the individual level and at home. It involves maintaining the cleanliness of our body and clothes. Personal hygiene is personal, as its name implies. In this regard, personal hygiene is defined as a condition promoting sanitary practices to the self. Everybody has their own habits and standards that they have been taught or that they have learned from others. Generally, the practice of personal hygiene is employed to prevent or minimize the incidence and spread of communicable diseases.

The exercise of proper personal hygiene is one of the essential parts of our daily life. Many people in rural areas may not understand what good or bad personal hygiene is. The prevention of communicable diseases, like diarrhea, trachoma and many others is highly possible through the application of proper personal hygiene. You need to learn the proper practice of personal hygiene and use this for the prevention and control of important public health diseases that are prevalent in your locality. This study session will also help you to understand the links between personal hygiene and one's dignity, confidence and comfort.

Health and Hygiene Cycle

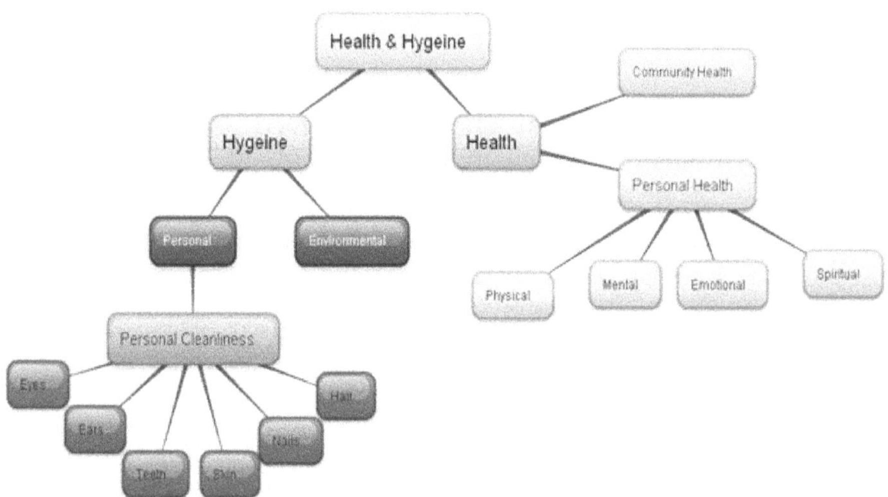

Health and Hygiene are essential parts of our daily life. Hygiene contains two basic elements

(a) Personal Hygiene
(b) Environmental Hygiene

Personal hygiene is keeping our body, our teeth, our hair, our clothes and our genital area clean. It is one of the mechanisms used for breaking disease transmission cycles. It also helps the individual to have a good aesthetic value by the people he/she is living with. Moreover, it is a good figure of better living style.

Personal hygiene is therefore, a measure taken at individual level to promote personal cleanliness so that transmission of diseases from source to susceptible hosts is prevented. It can be seen the most effective in protecting the health of communities where treatment options are constraints due to lack of health care delivery systems. Many health problems are due to poor hygiene behaviour. The benefits of safe water supply and sanitation efforts in a given community can easily be lost if the communities still carry on with the poor personal hygiene behaviour.

Health extension programs, such as Community Health and Personal health should consider carefully, so that the changes in hygiene practices and improve water and sanitation facilities. To achieve these goals, hygiene education and awareness plays a central role and has to be applied on a sustainable way.

The environmental health extension worker should focus on the following areas with respect to health information to better understand the importance of personal hygiene:

(a) The causative agents
(b) The mode of transmission
(c) Early diagnosis and treatment of cases
(d) Prevention and sanitary control measures

Disease transmission commonly occurs as a result of unhygienic disposal of human and household waste combined with poor hygienic practices.

Therefore, the fight against diseases requires:

(a) Recognition of microscopic forms of life
(b) Establishing microbes cause a specific disease
(c) Knowledge of methods of transmission of the disease
(d) Methods to fight the disease by applying different intervention like personal hygiene.

Some good practices should be followed in daily life such as

(a) Microbial and bacteria can also be a hazard to health when they are transferred from workers' hands onto food, cigarettes etc. and so taken into the body. This can be avoided by good personal hygiene, e.g. by: washing hands and face before eating, drinking and smoking and before, as well as after, using the toilet; eating, drinking and smoking only away from the work area.
(b) In cases where clothing may become contaminated, people should change out of this clothing before eating and drinking.

(c) Make sure those at risk know the hazards. Provide good washing facilities and somewhere clean to eat meals. Good clean welfare facilities can play an important part in protecting the health of everyone involved in the work.

(d) Make sure as few people as possible are exposed to hazardous substances by excluding people not directly involved in the work from the contaminated area.

Hygiene practices can reduce the risk of toxic materials being absorbed by workers or carried home to their families. Personal hygiene can help in breaking the disease transmission cycle.

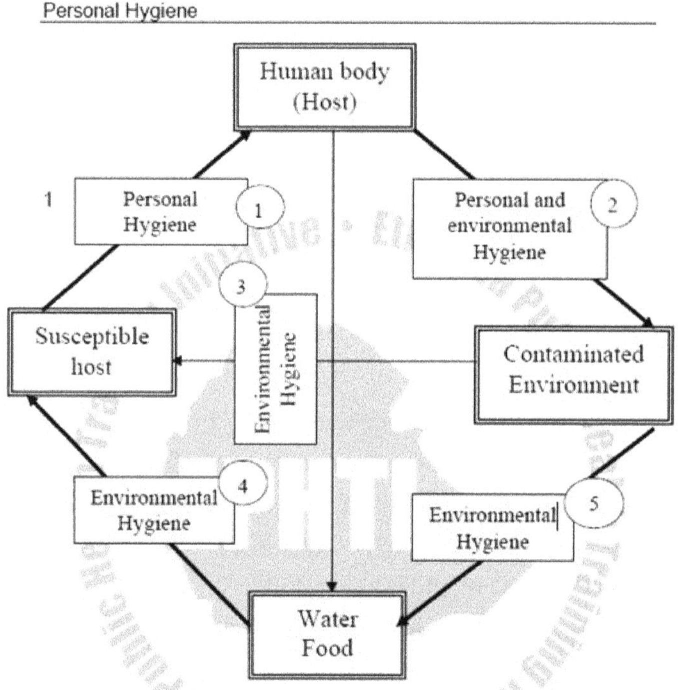

Fig 2.1 Mode of Transmission of disease and contamination from unhygienic person and environment

In the cycle, emphasis has been shown how contamination from one environment to the other environment like water and to human can happen. On the other side the diagram also shows where to apply a personal hygiene and environmental hygiene to interrupt or cut the vicious cycle for disease causation.

It is responsibility to change in hygienic behaviour in a given community has occurred in the direction desirable to promote healthy life style. The recognition of existing poor hygienic behaviour is the first step in developing hygiene education aimed at reducing sanitation related diseases in a particular community. Hygiene education should aim at encouraging the target community to be interested in having cleaner home, cleaner surrounding, cleaner neighborhood and cleaner environment through a greater understanding of why such cleanliness is necessary. It is only when such understanding is growing those sanitation efforts can succeed in making a difference and become sustainable.

2.2 Hair

Hair care is an overall term for parts of hygiene and cosmetology involving the hair on the human head. Hair care will differ according to one's hair type and according to various processes that can be applied to hair. All hair is not the same; hair is a manifestation of human diversity.

Biological Processes and Hygiene

Care of the hair and care of the scalp skin may appear separate, but are actually intertwined because hair grows from beneath the skin. The living parts of hair (hair follicle, hair root, root sheath, and sebaceous gland) are beneath the skin, while the actual hair shaft which emerges (the cuticle which covers the cortex and medulla) has no living processes. Damage or changes made to the visible hair shaft cannot be repaired by a biological process, though much can be done to manage hair and ensure that the cuticle remains intact.

Scalp skin, just like any other skin on the body, must be kept healthy to ensure a healthy body and healthy hair production. If the scalp is cleaned regularly by those who have rough hair or have a hair-fall problem, it can result in loss of hair. However, not all scalp disorders are a result of bacterial infections. Some arise inexplicably, and often only the symptoms can be treated for management of the condition (example: dandruff). There are also bacteria that can affect the hair itself. Head lice is probably the most common hair and scalp ailment worldwide. Head lice can be removed with great attention to detail, and studies show it is not necessarily associated with poor hygiene. More recent studies reveal that head lice actually thrive in clean hair. In this way, hair washing as a term may be a bit misleading, as what is necessary in healthy hair production and maintenance is often simply cleaning the surface of the scalp skin, the way the skin all over the body requires cleaning for good hygiene.

The sebaceous glands in human skin produce sebum, which is composed primarily of fatty acids. Sebum acts to protect hair and skin, and can inhibit the growth of microorganisms on the skin. Sebum contributes to the skin's slightly acidic natural pH somewhere between 5 and 6.8 on the pH spectrum. This oily substance gives hair moisture and shine as it travels naturally down the hair shaft, and serves as a protective substance preventing the hair from drying out or absorbing excessive amounts of external substances. Sebum is also distributed down the hair shaft "mechanically" by brushing and combing. When sebum is present in excess, the roots of the hair can appear oily, greasy, and darker than normal, and the hair may stick together.

Hair Cleaning

One way to distribute the hair's natural oils through the hair is by brushing with a natural bristle brush. The natural bristles effectively move the oil from the scalp through to the hair's mid-lengths and ends, nourishing these parts of the hair. Brushing the scalp also stimulates the sebaceous gland, which in turn produces more sebum. When sebum and sweat combine on the scalp surface, they help to create the acid mantle, which is the skin's own protective layer. Washing hair removes excess sweat and oil, as well as unwanted products from the hair and scalp.

Often hair is washed as part of a shower or bathing with shampoo, a specialized surfactant. Shampoos work by applying water and shampoo to the hair. The shampoo breaks the surface tension of the water, allowing the hair to become soaked. This is known as the wetting action. The wetting action is caused by the head of the shampoo molecule attracting the water to the hair shaft. Conversely, the tail of the shampoo molecule is attracted to the grease, dirt and oil on the hair shaft. The physical action of shampooing makes the grease and dirt become an emulsion that is then rinsed away with the water. This is known as the emulsifying action. Sulfate free shampoos are less harming on color treated hair than normal shampoos that contain sulfates. Sulfates strip away natural oils as well as hair dye. Sulfates are also responsible for the foaming effect of shampoos.

Shampoos have a pH of between 4 and 6 and do not contain soap. Sapless shampoos are acidic and therefore closer to the natural pH of hair. Acidic shampoos are the most common type used and maintain or improve the condition of the hair as they don't swell the hair shaft and don't strip the natural oils. Conditioners are often used after shampooing to smooth down the cuticle layer of the hair, which can become roughened during the physical process of shampooing. There are three main types of conditioners: anti-oxidant conditioners, which are mainly used in salons after chemical services and prevent creeping oxidation; internal conditioners, which enter into the cortex of the hair and help improve the hair's internal condition (also known as treatments); and external conditioners, or everyday conditioners, which smooth down the cuticle layer, making the hair shiny, comb able and smooth. Conditioners can also provide a physical layer of protection for the hair against physical and environmental damage.

A Step-by-Step way to wash your hair

1. Always brush hair to loosen dirt and scalp flakes, while activating oil glands.
2. Massage scalp gently to relieve tension and aid blood circulation in the scalp.
3. Wet hair thoroughly with warm or lukewarm water.
4. Pour a small amount of shampoo onto the palm of your hand, rub both hands together and smooth shampoo on evenly. (Pouring shampoo directly onto the hair makes even distribution impossible).
5. Massage shampoo into scalp with fingertips, adding more water for suds.
6. Spread the lather quickly throughout your hair, leave on for several seconds, comb through, and then rinse with warm water.
7. After the first thorough rinsing, the second rinse should be with water which is progressively colder. This reduces "swelling" of the hair tube and stimulates circulation. Cold water also makes the hairs stiffer and stronger, while locking them more firmly into their root.
8. The final step is to gently comb the hair with a wide-tooth comb rather than a brush which can stretch and break your hair.

Healthy Hair vs. Damaged Hair

HEALTHY HAIR
The hair is protected by the intact cuticle, sealing in moisture and natural oils. This helps to maintain strong hair.

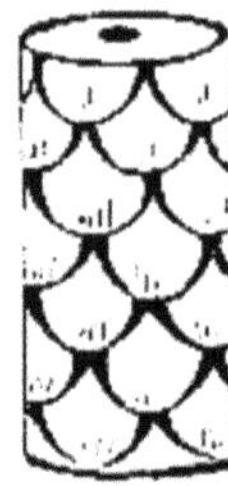

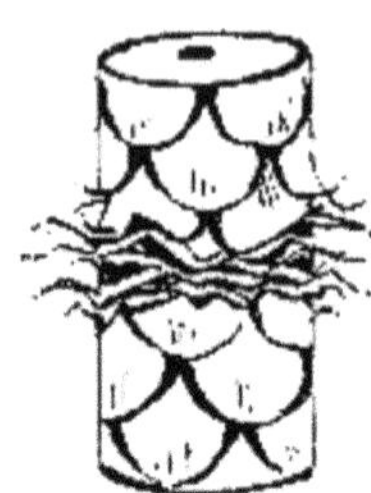

DAMAGED HAIR
The loss of moisture and natural oils makes hair fibres more susceptible to damage

A Guide to Protecting Your Hair

- Avoid prolonged exposure to sunlight, water, sand and chlorine.
- Cover your head with a hat as much as possible.
- In choosing a hair care product, look for ingredients that contain the following:

Aloe Vera to restore the precious moisture balance lost through blow-drying, tints and perms. Panthenol (Provitamin B5) protects hair from the damaging effects of the sun and pollutants. Jojoba Oil dissolves salt build-up due to perspiration.

EDTA removes chlorine damage caused by swimming pools and hot tubs.

2.3 Teeth and Mouth

Teeth are the only 25% of our whole mouth, it is made up of gums, tounge and cheeks as well. It has been found that unhealthy teets can lead to many diseases.

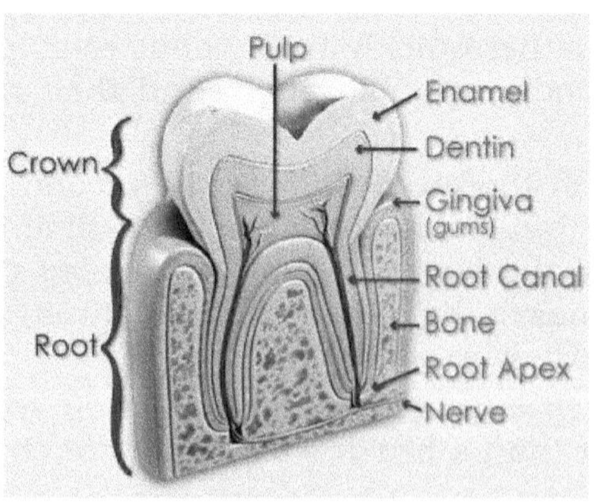

Care should be taken

Rinse after sugary foods. Food remnants feeds the bacteria in your mouth, which then excrete acidic substances that corrode tooth enamel, resulting in bad breath and painful jaw diseases. Sugar is especially fatal, even in low concentrations found in fruits, because it is sugar exposure time, which harms, not the amount of sugar you consume.

Brushing

Brush your teeth thoroughly at least twice a day, for two minutes each time. Make sure you brush on all sides of your teeth and get your tongue. You can ask your dentist(s) for a demonstration. It is best to do one of these times before you go to bed, as your mouth does not have the same salivary protection when you are sleeping as it does during the day. If you can, brush after lunch as well without toothpaste. Using lots of toothpaste may also discolour your teeth due to the fluoride content. Brushing during the day will reduce the damage caused by plaque by-products and toxins

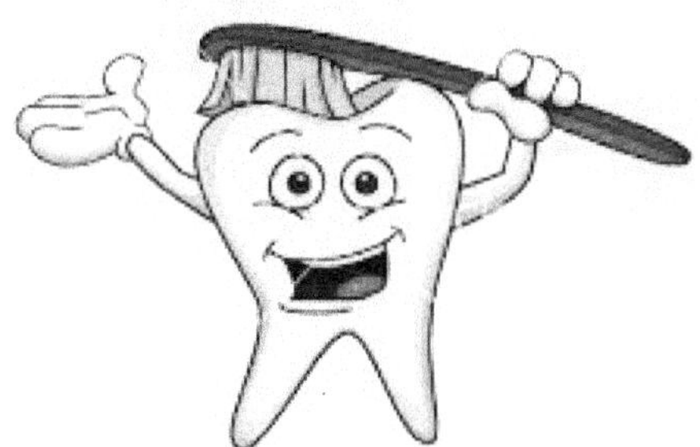

Bristle of Brush

Use a dry bristle brush for the first two minutes of cleaning. It's not the toothpaste that "cleans" your teeth, it's the mechanical action of the bristles toothpaste that "cleans" your teeth, it's the mechanical action of the bristles you can do a magnificent job brushing your teeth using a dry brush and rinsing with water (although your teeth will not have the benefit of fluoride). Also use a soft or ultra-soft bristle brush. Hold it at the edge so that you do not apply a lot of pressure invariably.

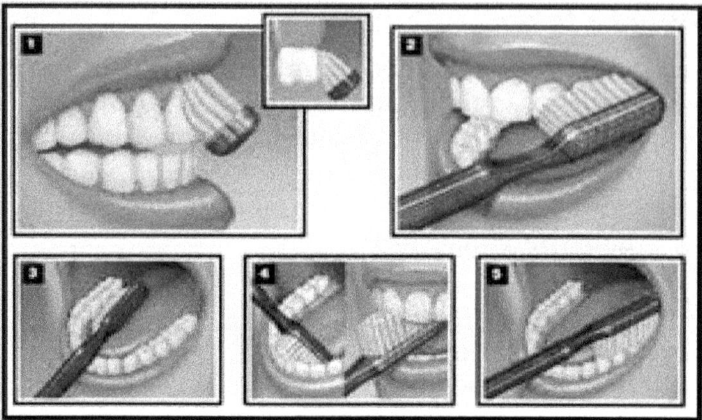

Floss

Floss your teeth daily and after any food that will stick in your teeth (i.e. corn on the cob, caramel, peanut butter, etc.). This cleans the other sides of your teeth that you couldn't reach with your toothbrush. Flossing is always done at night.

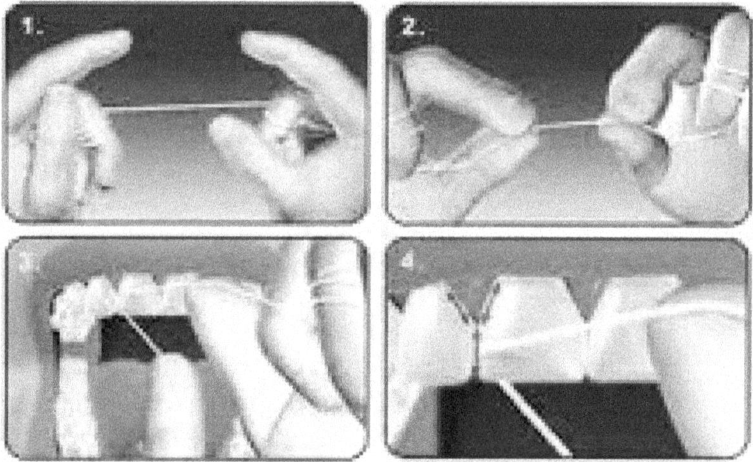

Tongue

Use a tongue scraper. A tongue scraper is an important part of oral hygiene that will also work wonders with stale, smelly breath. Use it to remove the plaque on your tongue, which will freshen breath and presumably slow down the accumulation of plaque on your teeth. Alternatively, you can use your toothbrush to clean your tongue.

Mouthwash

Find a fluoride mouthwash. Fluoride mouthwashes help to strengthen tooth enamel. Teach children between the age of six and twelve good rinsing skills to prevent swallowing. Follow the directions on the bottle. Right before you got to bed is a good time.

Dentist

Visit your dentist at least every six months and every time that you have a problem with your teeth. Schedule a professional cleaning with a registered dental hygienist. Be an "informed health care consumer" and pay attention to what is going on. Ask your dental hygienist what your probing are at each visit

Tips to remember

1. Don't forget to brush the back of your tongue and the upper palate of your mouth
2. Try to drink milk, as it is high in calcium. Calcium helps bones and teeth to grow stronger.
3. Use mouth wash after brushing.
4. Replace your toothbrush every three months.
5. After having an especially sugary drink, washing your mouth out with water or milk will help get rid of harmful acids?
6. Understand that when you brush, you don't need a lot of toothpaste; just squeeze out a bit the size of a pea.
7. Drink acidic beverages (such as juice and soda) with a straw. The liquid will not contact your teeth, and therefore, not decay the enamel. Tips don't forget to brush the back of your tongue and the upper palate of your mouth.
8. Try to drink milk, as it is high in calcium. Calcium helps bones and teeth to grow stronger.
9. When you use mouthwash, use as directed on the bottle, read all instructions BEFORE using the product.
10. Spend extra time on the back teeth along the gum-line, gums, as plaque and other bacteria can build up easily there because of your saliva stream

Mouth

Dry Mouth

Dry mouth happens when you don't have enough saliva, or spit, to keep your mouth wet. Many common medicines can cause dry mouth. That can make it hard to eat, swallow, taste, and even speak. Dry mouth can cause tooth decay and other infections of the mouth.

There are some things you can try that may help with dry mouth. Try sipping water or sugarless drinks. Don't smoke and avoid alcohol and caffeine. Sugarless hard candy or sugarless gum may help. Your dentist or doctor might suggest that you use artificial saliva to keep your mouth wet. Or they may have other ideas on how to cope with dry mouth.

Oral Cancer

Cancer of the mouth can grow in any part of the mouth or throat. It is more likely to happen in people over age 40. A dental check-up is a good time for your dentist to look for signs of oral cancer. Pain is not usually an early symptom of the disease. Treatment works best before the disease spreads. Even if you have lost all your natural teeth, you should still see your dentist for regular oral cancer exams.

You can lower your risk of getting oral cancer in a few ways:

- Do not use tobacco products - cigarettes, chewing tobacco, snuff, pipes, or cigars
- If you drink alcohol, do so only in moderation
- Use lip balm with sunscreen

2.4 Skin

Introduction

The skin is the largest organ of the body, with a total area of about 20 square feet. The skin protects us from microbes and the elements, helps regulate body temperature, and permits the sensations of touch, heat, and cold.

Skin has three layers:

- The epidermis, the outermost layer of skin, provides a waterproof barrier and creates our skin tone.

- The dermis, beneath the epidermis, contains tough connective tissue, hair follicles, and sweat glands.
- The deeper subcutaneous tissue (hypodermis) is made of fat and connective tissue.

The skin's colour is created by special cells called melanocytes, which produce the pigment melanin. Melanocytes are located in the epidermis.

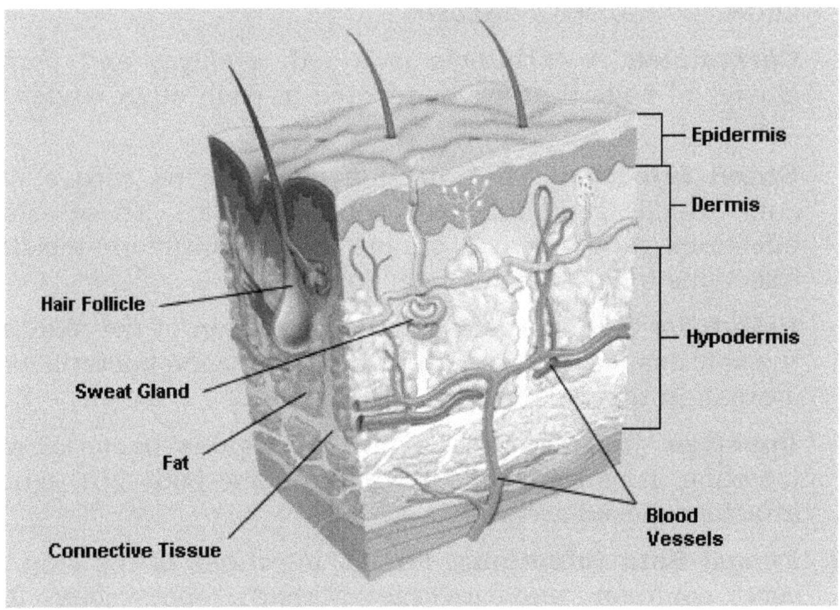

Importance of Skin Hygiene

Proper skin hygiene is important because unclean skin favours the development of pathogenic organisms. The dead cells that continually slough off the epidermis mix with the secretions of the sweat and sebaceous glands and the dust found on the skin form a filthy layer on its surface. If not washed away, the slurry of sweat and sebaceous secretions mixed with dirt and dead skin is decomposed by bacterial flora, producing a foul smell. Functions of the skin are disturbed when it is excessively dirty; it becomes more easily damaged, the release of antibacterial compounds decreases and dirty skin is more prone to develop infections. Cosmetics should be used carefully on the skin because these may cause allergic reactions.

Causes of Poor Skin Hygiene

The following medical conditions are some of the possible causes of Poor skin hygiene.

Basically skin infections are of three types they are as follows:

1. **Bacterial Skin Infections:**

   Leprosy: Leprosy is caused by a slow-growing type of bacteria called Mycobacteriumleprae. Leprosy is also known as Hansen's disease.

   Carbuncles: A carbuncle is a red, swollen, and painful cluster of boils that are connected to each other under the skin.

   Staph Infection: The infection often begins with a little cut, which gets infected with bacteria. These staph infections range from a simple boil to antibiotic-resistant infections to flesh-eating infections.

   Cellulitis: Cellulitis is a common infection of the skin and the soft tissues underneath. It happens when bacteria enter a break in the skin and spread.

   Impetigo: Impetigo is a highly contagious bacterial skin infection. It can appear anywhere on the body but usually attacks exposed areas.

2. **Fungal Skin Infections:** Fungal infections of the skin are very common and include athlete's foot, jock itch, ringworm, and yeast infections.

   Ringworm: Worms don't cause ringworm. Rather, this superficial skin infection, also known as tinea, is caused by fungi called dermatophytes.

   Athlete's Foot: Athlete's foot is a common fungal infection and you don't have to be an athlete to get it. This annoying ailment occurs in boys, girls, men, and women of all ages.

   Candidiasis (Yeast Infection): Candidiasis is an infection caused by a group of yeast. There are more than 20 species of Candida, the most common being Candida albicans. These fungi live on all surfaces of our bodies.

   Fungal Nail Infections: A fungal nail infection occurs when a fungus attacks a fingernail, a toenail, or the skin under the nail, called the nail bed.

3. Viral Skin Infections

Molluscum Contagiosum: Molluscum contagiosum is a viral skin infection that causes either single or multiple raised, pearl-like bumps (papules) on the skin.

Chickenpox: Chickenpox (varicella), a viral illness characterized by a very itchy red rash, is one of the most common infectious diseases of childhood.

Four Steps for a Healthy Skin:

1. *Cleansing*: Find a good Cleanser that your skin responds well to, and stick with it. Choose a Creamy Cleanser if you have dry skin or a Clear Cleanser if you have oily skin. Be careful not to cleanse too often, you risk over-cleansing skin, you really only need to wash your face at night to remove makeup and sunscreen, which can clog pores. If you have dry skin, consider cold cream. Use warm water to loosen dirt and clogged pores. Use a dime-sized bit of cleanser, and then rinse with cool or lukewarm water. In the morning, a splash of lukewarm water is all you need. Never wash your face with hot or cold water (both can cause broken capillaries).
2. *Exfoliation*: If you start properly exfoliating your skin, you will notice an almost immediate difference. Put a dab of cleanser on a damp washcloth and massage the cleanser into my skin in a circular motion. After a quick rinse, any sign of dead skin is erased. You can also exfoliate skin via microdermabrasion, chemical peels and Retinoids. Scrubs work by removing the top layer of dead skin cells that tend to dull your complexion. Make sure you use a gentle scrub with tiny grains. Big grains in cheap scrubs can tear skin and cause more harm than good. Retinoids also work by removing the top layer of dead skin cells while also generating collagen in the skin. Skincare experts consider Retinoids to be a miracle skin saver.
3. *Moisturizing*: If you have dry skin, you should invest in a Basic Moisturizer. How much should you moisturize? Your skin will tell you. When your skin is tight, it's crying out for moisture. Be careful not to over-moisturize, this can close pores.

4. *Sun Screen*: Major cause of wrinkles is sun damage, so it's important to use a sunscreen of at least 30 SPF from your early years on even in winter and on cloudy days. A great trick is to purchase two moisturizers: One for night and one for day that includes UV protection. Don't use moisturizers with sunscreen at night; make sure it contains Mexoryl or Helioplex.

2.5 Hands

A hand is a prehensile, multi-fingered extremity located at the end of an arm or forelimb of humans. The human hand has 27 bones, not including the sesamoid bone, the number of which varies between people, 14 of which are the phalanges (proximal, intermediate and distal) of the fingers.

Areas of the human hand include:

- **The palm**, which is the central region of the anterior part of the hand, located superficially to the metacarpus. The skin in this area contains dermal papillae to increase friction, such as are also present on the fingers and used for fingerprints.
- **The opisthenar area** (dorsal) is the corresponding area on the posterior part of the hand.
- **The heel of the hand** is the area anteriorly to the bases of the metacarpal bones, located in the proximal part of the palm. It is the area that sustains most pressure when using the palm of the hand for support, such as in handstand.

There are five digits attached to the hand. The four fingers can be folded over the palm which allows the grasping of objects. Each finger, starting with the one closest to the thumb, has a colloquial name to distinguish it from the others

- Index finger, pointer finger, or forefinger
- Middle finger or long finger,
- Ring finger
- Little finger, pinkie finger, or small finger.

The thumb (connected to the trapezium) is located on one of the sides, parallel to the arm. A reliable way of identifying human hands is from the presence of opposable thumbs.

Opposable thumbs are identified by the ability to be brought opposite to the fingers, a muscle action known as opposition.

Hygiene for Hands

Hands are one of the most used physical part of body, to touch, to do work, to eat, to clean etc...So while doing all these things tidiness is to be maintained otherwise diseases occur. Even W.H.O have started a campaign to create awareness on cleaning hand before doing certain works which even saves lives of people at certain circumstances. Because hands touch all the parts of your body and touch all the physically fallen objects they should be cleaned periodically. According to the act to be done (like eating, treatment etc.) washing hands with soap is recommended.

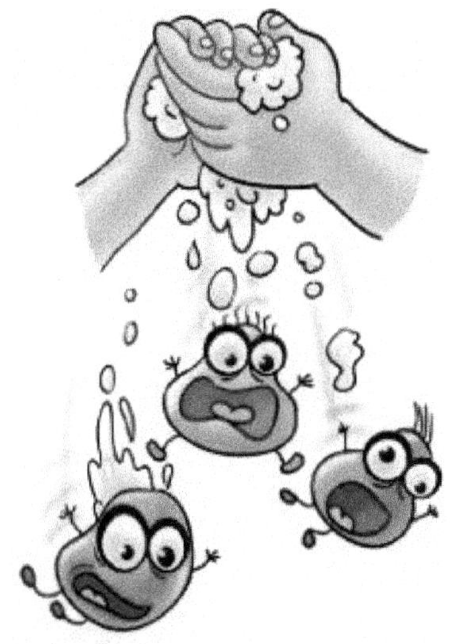

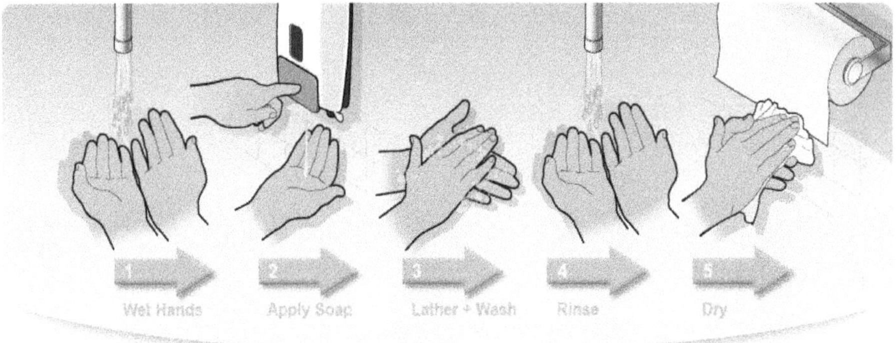

If soap is not available then just rinse your hands with water as shown in the picture below.

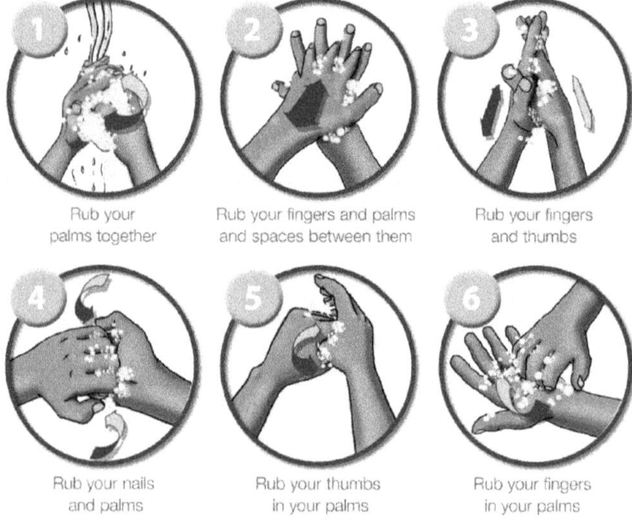

Nails

Nails are very important parts of our hands. Cleaning your nails without any dirt and cutting your nails time to time will keep you out of diseases.

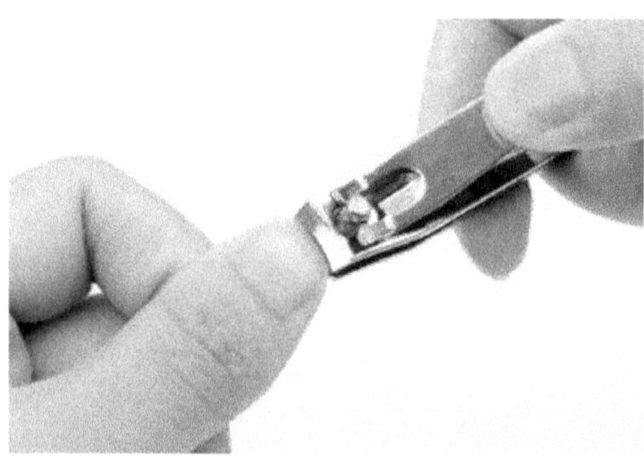

2.6 Feet

Maintaining good foot hygiene is an important part of personal care. By taking care of your feet, you can prevent fungal infections like athlete's foot and other common foot ailments that affect so many people. All you need to do is spend a few minutes every day cleaning and caring for your feet. Your reward will be a higher sense of personal comfort and confidence, and also feet that look and smell great.

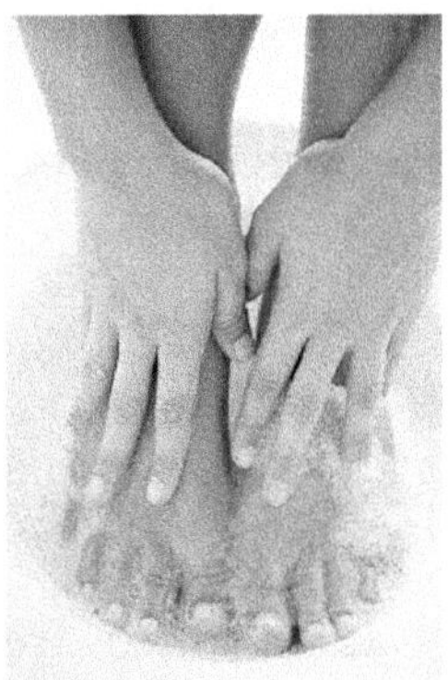

- It is important to clean your feet every day with warm water and soap.
- Avoid harsh soaps that irritate the skin and strip it of moisture.
- Hot water must also be avoided for the same reason. Scrub gently, and wash thoroughly.
- Take the time to scrub between your toes as well.

Dry you're Feet

- Use a towel to dry your feet thoroughly.
- Avoid sharing your soap or towel with anybody else.
- Tuck the towel between your toes and dry the skin.
- Avoid wearing close fitting footwear till your feet at totally dry

Wear Cotton Socks

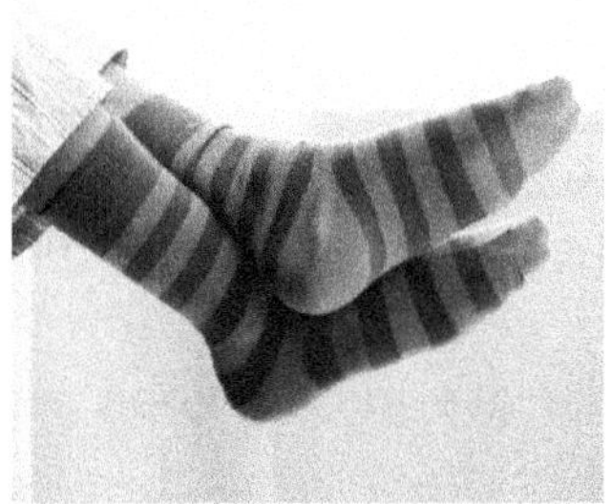

- Avoid synthetic material on your feet, as they restrict the flow of air.
- Cotton or woollen socks are the best choices, as they let your skin breathe. These materials are also absorptive, which makes the sweat more manageable.
- Choose footwear that you are comfortable in. If your shoes are too tight, your feet will sweat more.
- This makes the feet more susceptible to fungal and bacterial attacks.

Air Your Feet Regularly

- When possible, remove your footwear and expose your feet to the air.
- This simple action is vital to freshening your feet and reducing the risk of any infections.
- When constantly covered, feet are more susceptible to several problems like smell, dampness, and itchiness.

Keep Your Toenails Short

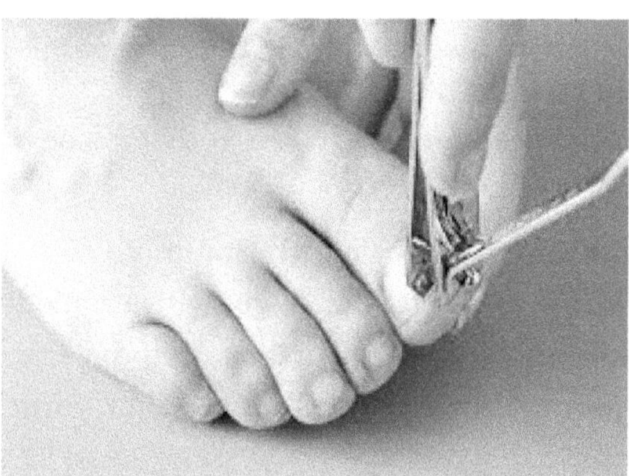

- Maintain your toenails. Use a nail clipper to keep them short and clean.
- This reduces the risk of ingrown toenails, which can be a painful condition.
- Keeping toenails clean is also an important part of personal hygiene.
- Regular pedicures are also a good way of maintaining the health of your feet.

Inspect Your Feet Regularly

- As with other conditions, prevention of foot ailments is better than cure.
- Regular inspection of your feet will alert you to calluses, swelling, blistering, cuts, and blisters.
- These small conditions, if left untreated, can cause much more severe problems later.
- Exfoliate and Moisturize
- Soak your feet in warm water and use a pumice stone or exfoliating brush to scrub your feet.
- This will remove any hard, dry skin and keep the feet soft.
- Follow up with a mild moisturizer to keep your skin moist.
- Regular exfoliation will prevent the formation of cracked heels and calluses on your feet.

2.7 Nose and Eyes

Nose

The nose is an important part of our body which allows us to enjoy that smells of the world. Allergies colds and other problems can cause the nose to function at less than its best. The nose serves two purposes. It provides an avenue for smelling which increases pleasure, warns against danger, and helps to improve the quality of life. It also serves as an airway into the lungs. A healthy nose will help filter particles from the airway much better than an unhealthy nose will. A chronically runny nose or stuffy nose can lead to headaches and other discomfort as well as become an irritating source of discomfort on its own.

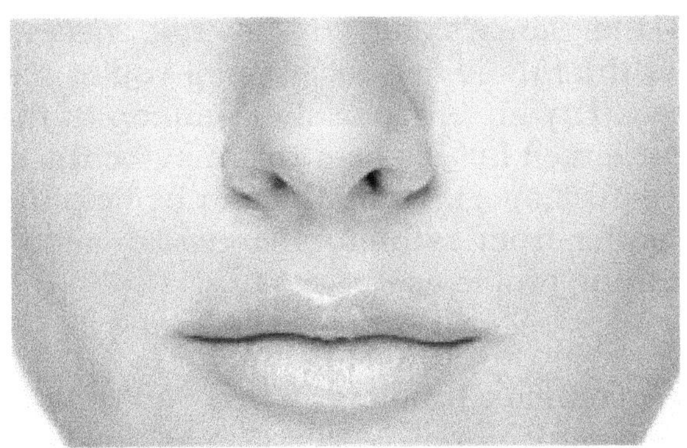

Care of Your Nose

There are many things that we subject our noses to that are unhealthy and problematic for healthy breathing. Learning how to take care of your nose can help you enjoy a pain free, symptom free, lifelong experience of some of the world's most tantalizing smells. Your nose and sinuses are intimately connected, and helping to improve your nose health will help you to improve sinus health.

While nasal sprays are an obvious solution to nasal problems, they don't necessarily induce good nose health. In fact, many sprays are targeting your sinuses and not your nose, and thus can be damaging or irritating to the lining along the nostrils. If you do have to use a nasal spray, be sure to follow the directions and avoid spraying any more than absolutely necessary. Never exceed the dosing instructions or take it longer than prescribed as this can lead to serious problems.

Warm steam

Warm steam breathed in through the nostrils can actually help more than sprays. If you inhale the steam between 4 and 6 times daily without an additive, you can often help clear up sinuses and improve your nasal passages quickly without the risk of harming membranes.

Humidity in the Air

Keeping your home's air a bit more humid can help improve nose health as well. Humidity helps prevent things like waking in the middle of the night with nasal problems and can increase the ease of breathing. In some cases it can also help cut down on snoring because the nasal passages are not clogged.

Using a simple humidifier will allow you to control the level of moisture in the home's air. It is not necessary to add medications to the humidifier because all you're seeking is relief from the dry air. Dry air is especially common in the winter time and if you have forced hot air heat this may be the only time that you experience discomfort. Humidity can be helpful regardless of whether you suffer from asthma, allergies, or tend not to suffer from any breathing problems.

Allergens

Allergens are a common problem. When you're taking good care of your nose you want to relieve allergies as quickly and easily as possible while minimizing the need for medications. Allergy medications tend to dry the nasal passages too much, make one sleepy, or keep one awake at night. Thus, the more you can do to eliminate household allergens and other triggers the better off you are.

Air filtration can be beneficial for helping your nose stay happy and healthy. Nasal allergies can be very difficult to live with and keeping a filtration system in top working order can help improve the situation. You also want to make sure that you clean or replace the air filter in your heating and cooling units regularly.

Vacuum cleaners with filters should be kept at top filtration capacity. Many people with allergies do better in homes with hard floors instead of carpeting because there are fewer fibres to trap dander, mites, and dust. If you need help controlling allergies see your physician and ask about alternatives to medication. The severity of your nasal allergies will determine how many natural options you might have.

Keeping nose clean

A cleaner nose is a happier nose. The way you clean your nose is important. To take care of your nose properly you will want to make sure that it receives the same kind of care that you want your skin and hair to have. With a cotton swab and warm, mildly salty water you can clean your nose without risk of scratching or cutting and you will not damage the sensitive membranes.

With mildly salted warm water on a cotton swab you will want to clean any debris from the nose without going far up into the nasal passages. Ultimately, you want to avoid sticking anything in your nose, but for cleaning purposes this is often the safest and most effective method. Cleaning your nose not only helps to keep it comfortable but it also helps to improve its ability to filter particles. Cleaner noses tend to develop fewer allergic reactions and help to reduce snoring as well. Thus, you want to make sure that you maintain a clean and healthy nose as part of your daily routine.

Smoking injuries to nose

Cigarette smoking is damaging. The nasal cavity suffers more from smoking menthol cigarettes than it does from non-menthol cigarettes. Pipes, cigars, and other forms of smoking can also cause irritation and damage to the lining of the nasal passages. If you can avoid smoking altogether, you are helping your nose avoid long term dryness, irritation, and sensitivity to allergen triggers. You are also saving your life.

Of course, avoiding second hand smoke and other pollutants will help reduce the risk of damage to the membranes as well. You will want to breathe the cleanest air possible. If you smoke, you're not going to be able to feel the benefits as fully when it comes to taking care of your nose.

The more you do to learn how to take care of your nose the easier breathing will be. Clear from debris and allergens your nasal passages can relax. Inflammation can often be caused by triggers other than allergies. This means that once the inflammation is gone the allergen triggers may not be nearly as intense. Healthy noses and happy breathing is part of living healthier lives.

Eyes

Human Eye

The human eye is an organ that reacts to light and has several purposes. As a sense organ, the mammalian eye allows vision. Rod and cone cells in the retina allow conscious light perception and vision including colour differentiation and the perception of depth. The human eye can distinguish about 10 million colours.

Structure of an eye

The eye is not shaped like a perfect sphere, rather it is a fused two-piece unit. The smaller frontal unit, transparent and more curved, called the cornea is linked to the larger white unit called the sclera. The corneal segment is typically about 8 mm (0.3 in) in radius. The sclerotic chamber constitutes the remaining five-sixths; its radius is typically about 12 mm. The cornea and sclera are connected by a ring called the limbs. The iris is the collared circular structure concentrically surrounding the centre of the eye, the pupil, which appears to be black. To see inside the eye, a device known as an ophthalmoscope is used.

Size

The dimensions differ among adults by only one or two millimetres; it is remarkably consistent across different ethnicities. The vertical measure, generally less than the horizontal distance, is about 24 mm among adults, at birth about 16–17 millimetres (about 0.65 inch). The transverse size of a human adult eye is approximately 24.2 mm and the sagittal size is 23.7 mm with no significant difference between sexes and age groups. The eyeball grows rapidly, increasing to 22.5–23 mm (approx. 0.89 in) by three years of age. By age 13, the eye attains its full size. The typical adult eye has an anterior to posterior diameter of 24 millimetres, a volume of six cubic centimetres (0.4 cu. in.), and a mass of 7.5 grams.

Anatomy of the human eye

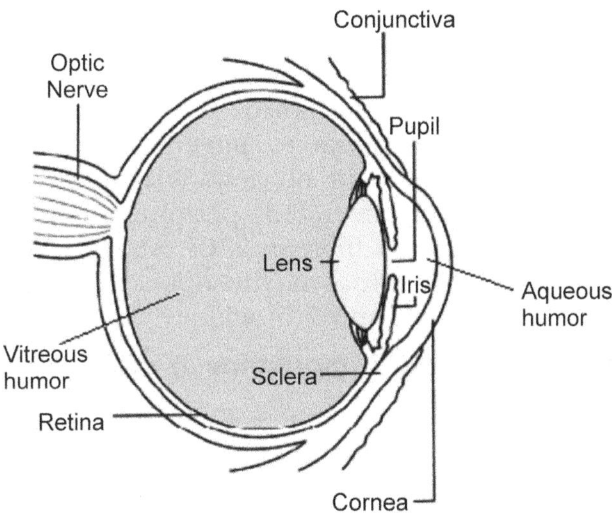

Cornea: the transparent part at the front of the eye that refracts light entering the eye onto the lens.

Lens: a transparent structure behind the pupil that refracts incoming light and focuses it onto the retina. The lens is able to change shape in order to improve the focus.

Iris: This is the coloured part of the eye that controls the amount of light that enters the eye, it is able to contact and dilate in order to control the size of the pupil depending on the light intensity. Sclera: the outer white part of the eye that protects the inner structures.

Retina: This is the light sensitive layer inside the eye that contains light sensitive photoreceptive cells called rods and cones. These cells change light into sight by converting light into electrical impulses. These electrical messages are sent from the retina to the brain and interpreted as images.

Optic nerve: This leaves the eye at the optic disk and transfers all the visual information to the brain.

Conjunctiva: A transparent vascular membrane that lines the inside of the eyelids and extends over the front of the white part of the eye (the sclera).

Aqueous humour: This fluid circulates the front part of the eye, it provides nourishment and helps maintain the eye pressure.

Vitreous humour: The clear gel in the centre of the eye that helps the eye to maintain its spherical shape.

Field of view

The approximate field of view of an individual human eye is 95° away from the nose, 75° downward, 60° toward the nose, and 60° upward, allowing humans to have an almost 180-degree forward-facing horizontal field of view. With eyeball rotation of about 90° (head rotation excluded, peripheral vision included), horizontal field of view is as high as 270°. About 12–15° temporal and 1.5° below the horizontal is the optic nerve or blind spot which is roughly 7.5° high and 5.5° wide

What is eye hygiene and importance of eye hygiene?

Every day we submit our eyes to a multitude of environmental factors. Eyes are in constant contact with air pollutants, bacteria, dry air, wind, cosmetics and many other factors. Eyelashes and eyelids give a certain amount of protection but it is often not sufficient for sensitive areas of the eye. Environmental factors can be the cause of lid infections, which in some cases may be the cause of secretions, flaking or crusting.

Eye Hygiene Methods

Normally, your eyes get cleaned sufficiently by simply washing your face. If you have a tendency to oily skin, dandruff and lid crusting it is recommended that you also carry out extensive lid hygiene on a daily basis to prevent infections of the lid. The eyelid has sebaceous glands, which can sometimes become blocked. This can cause unpleasant infections. To help prevent this - once a day gently massage the outside of the eyelids (eyes closed) with a hand towel (or cotton buds) soaked in warm water or a mild baby shampoo. By doing this you can control bacterial growth and massage the blocked lipids out of the glands. Equally important is the removal of all makeup and the cleansing of the eyes at the end of each day. Particles of makeup can otherwise get into your eyes during the night and cause irritation. When taking off your makeup always move the cotton pad inward toward your nose. If you rub in the other direction the lower lid can be pulled away slightly creating a pocket where debris can get in. Any types of hard and sharp particles can damage your cornea.

Eyelid hygiene

This factsheet will identify some of the problems people may have with eyelid and eyelash hygiene and some of the difficulties that can result from poor hygiene. It will offer some practical help to keep eyes clean.

1. Eyelids and eyelashes protect our eyes which can easily be damaged. It is important that eyelids and eyelashes are kept clean and healthy so people see clearly and avoid pain or discomfort.
2. The front on the eye (the sclera, cornea and conjunctiva) needs to be moist, smooth and clear at all times. Tears, which cover the cornea, remove dust and dirt particles from eyes. They also offer some protection against tiny invisible organisms which could cause damage.
3. Eyelids also prevent things getting on to the eye. Eyelids contain glands that secrete oils that travel from the glands through ducts and on to the eye. These oils help to prevent tears from evaporating.
4. The eyelids have eyelashes that grow out of the edge of the eyelid. This area is called the 'eyelid margin'. The eyelashes help to protect the eye by stopping things getting on to the Eye. Eyelashes also alert people to when something is too close to the eye.

Eyelid problems

Blocked glands or ducts in the eyelids can prevent the oils getting on to the eye. This means there will be no oil to stop the tears from evaporating. When tears evaporate too quickly it can lead to dry eyes. Dry eye can be uncomfortable and painful and can eventually lead to a reduction in vision. A bacteria called staphylococcus aurous is present on the eyelid skin and eyelid margin. This can make the eyelids inflamed, so they look red. Inflammation may make the eyelid feel itchy as well as be uncomfortable and painful.

Eyelid cleansing

With the consent of the person, eyelids may be kept clean and healthy as part of a daily routine. Cleaning of the eyelids can be made part of a person's daily routine, like having a wash in the bathroom wash-hand basin or having a shower. The supporter should follow strict hygiene guidelines, including hand and fingernail

Cleanliness and disposal of swabs or paper towels. Cross infection must be avoided. The aim of cleaning the eyelids is to remove the debris of dead skin cells and bacteria that can gather on the eyelids.

The following should be done to carry out external eyelid cleansing.

- Use sterile warm water in a small sterilised basin and mix in two or three drops of the 'non-sting' anti-allergenic shampoo solution.
- Dip the cotton end of a bud into the water/soap mixture. Gently move the soaked cotton bud along the front eyelid margin, where the eyelashes grow out of the eyelid. This may have to be repeated many times over in the one session.
- Always follow the advice given by a medical practitioner Always follow any procedure or recording that might be required

Besides cleaning your lids with cotton buds there are many other ways of keeping good eye hygiene:

Sterilised Eye Cleaning Pads

A relatively new product on the market - hygienic eye care pads. Each pad is individually packed to ensure sterile, hygienic cleansing of the eye; ideal for babies, children and adults. These pads are also used for removing makeup and flaking skin. These moistened pads are soaked in plant extracts. These soothe and cleanse the eye, reducing puffiness, providing moisture and coolness for tired and strained eyes.

Cleaning Gels

For good eye hygiene cleaning gels specially developed for the eyes are available in tubes. Some of the gel is placed on a paper tissue to cleanse the eye. Always check the expiry dates on gels and never touch the tube opening with your fingers - bacteria can easily be transferred from the tip of the tube to your eye.

Eye Baths

Eye baths are available for maintaining eye hygiene. Eye bath solutions with a special "eyetub" are available at your local chemist. These baths rinse and relieve eye irritations and dryness caused by computer work, reading, television and the like. Eye baths can also benefit those prone to allergies by rinsing out dust and pollen. Eye baths are often used in first aid to treat the incursion of foreign bodies or similar injuries to the eye. Always consult an ophthalmologist immediately in the event of damage to the eye.

Use care with Homemade Products

It is very important to be careful when using homemade products for the eye such as camomile rinses. Camomile has the reputation of having soothing effects and this is very true. However, based on latest research studies, camomile tends to have a drying effect on the eyes. Camomile also often contains pollen, which can prove problematic for those with allergies. And if the homemade solution has been sitting a while it may become an ideal environment for bacterial growth. When it comes to eye hygiene it is best to stick to tested products recommended by your chemist or ophthalmologist

Good eye hygiene practice also involves caring for the delicate skin around the eye. As we know this skin is very thin and not well padded making it susceptible to dryness and the development of fine lines. Many creams and gels recommended for sensitive eyes and contact lens wearers are available on the market. Take the time to try these out and to find out what products are best for you.

Eye irritation

Eye irritation has been defined as "the magnitude of any stinging, scratching, burning, or other irritating sensation from the eye. It is a common problem experienced by people of all ages. Related eye symptoms and signs of irritation are discomfort, dryness, excess tearing, itching, grating, sandy sensation, ocular fatigue, pain, scratchiness, soreness, redness, swollen eyelids, and tiredness, etc. These eye symptoms are reported with intensities from severe to mild. It has been suggested that these eye symptoms are related to different causal mechanisms.

Several suspected causal factors in our environment have been studied sofar. One hypothesis is that indoor air pollution may cause eye and airway irritation. Eye irritation depends somewhat on destabilization of the outer-eye tear film, in which the formation of dry spots result in such ocular discomfort as dryness. Occupational factors are also likely to influence the perception of eye irritation. Some of these are lighting (glare and poor contrast), gaze position, a limited number of breaks, and a constant function of accommodation, musculoskeletal burden, and impairment of the visual nervous system. Another factor that may be related is work stress other risk factors, such as chemical toxins/irritants (e.g. amines, formaldehyde, acetaldehyde, acrolein, N-decane, VOCs, ozone, pesticides and preservatives, allergens, etc.) might cause eye irritation as well.

Certain volatile organic compounds that are both chemically reactive and airway irritants may cause eye irritation. Personal factors (e.g. use of contact lenses, eye make-up, and certain medications) may also affect destabilization of the tear film and possibly result in more eye symptoms. Nevertheless, if airborne particles alone should destabilize the tear film and cause eye irritation, their content of surface-active compounds must be high. An integrated physiological risk model with blink frequency, destabilization, and break-up of the eye tear film as inseparable phenomena may explain eye irritation among office workers in terms of occupational, climate, and eye-related physiological risk factors.

There are other factors that are related to eye irritation as well. Three major factors that influence the most are indoor air pollution, contact lenses and gender differences. Field studies have found that the prevalence of objective eye signs is often significantly altered among office workers in comparisons with random samples of the general population. These research results might indicate that indoor air pollution has played an important role in causing eye irritation. There are more and more people wearing contact lens now and dry eyes appear to be the most common complaint among contact lens wearers. Although both contact lens wearers and spectacle wearers experience similar eye irritation symptoms, dryness, redness, and grittiness have been reported far more frequently among contact lens wearers and with greater severity than among spectacle wearers. Studies have shown that incidence of dry eyes increases with age. Especially among women. Tear film stability (e.g. break-up time) is significantly lower among women than among men. In addition, women have a higher blink frequency while reading. Several factors may contribute to gender differences. One is the use of eye make-up. Another reason could be that the women in the reported studies have done more VDU work than the men, including lower grade work. A third often-quoted explanation is related to the age-dependent decrease of tear secretion, particularly among women after 40 years of age.

In a study conducted by UCLA, the frequency of reported symptoms in industrial buildings was investigated. The study's results were that eye irritation was the most frequent symptom in industrial building spaces, at 81%. Modern office work with use of office equipment has raised concerns about possible adverse health effects. Since the 1970s, reports have linked mucosal, skin, and general symptoms to work with self-copying paper. Emission of various particulate and volatile substances has been suggested as specific causes. These symptoms have been related to Sick building syndrome (SBS), which involves symptoms such as irritation to the eyes, skin, and upper airways, headache and fatigue.

Many of the symptoms described in SBS and multiple chemical sensitivity (MCS) resemble the symptoms known to be elicited by airborne irritant chemicals. A repeated measurement design was employed in the study of acute symptoms of eye and respiratory tract irritation resulting from occupational exposure to sodium borate dusts. The symptom assessment of the 79 exposed and 27 unexposed subjects comprised interviews before the shift began and then at regular hourly intervals for the next six hours of the shift, four days in a row. Exposures were monitored concurrently with a personal real time aerosol monitor. Two different exposure profiles, a daily average and short term (15 minute) average, were used in the analysis. Exposure-response relations were evaluated by linking incidence rates for each symptom with categories of exposure.

Several actions can be taken to prevent eye irritation: Trying to maintain normal blinking by avoiding room temperatures that are too high; avoiding relative humidifies that are too high or too low, because they reduce blink frequency or may increase water evaporation

Defects of the Eye

Myopia: (near-sightedness) this is a defect of vision in which far objects appear blurred but near objects are seen clearly. The image is focused in front of the retina rather than on it usually because the eyeball is too long or the refractive power of the eye's lens too strong. Myopia can be corrected by wearing glasses/contacts with concave lenses these help to focus the image on the retina.

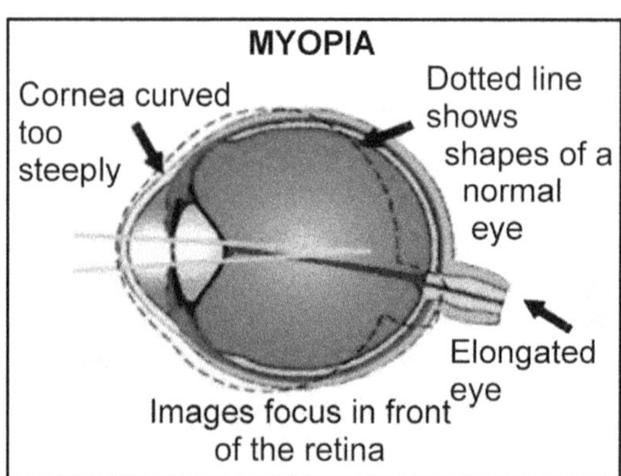

Hyperopia: (farsightedness) this is a defect of vision in which there is difficulty with near vision but far objects can be seen easily. The image is focused behind the retina rather than upon it. This occurs when the eyeball is too short or the refractive power of the lens is too weak.

Hyperopia can be corrected by wearing glasses/contacts that contain convex lenses.

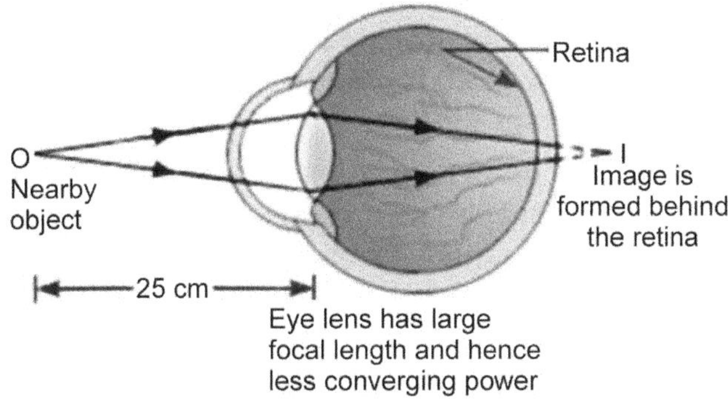

Astigmatism: This defect is when the light rays do not all come to a single focal point on the retina, instead some focus on the retina and some focus in front of or behind it. This is usually caused by a non-uniform curvature of the cornea. A typical symptom of astigmatism is if you are looking at a pattern of lines placed at various angles and the lines running in one direction appear sharp whilst those in other directions appear blurred. Astigmatism can usually be corrected by using a special spherical cylindrical lens; this is placed in the out-of-focus axis.

Astigmatism

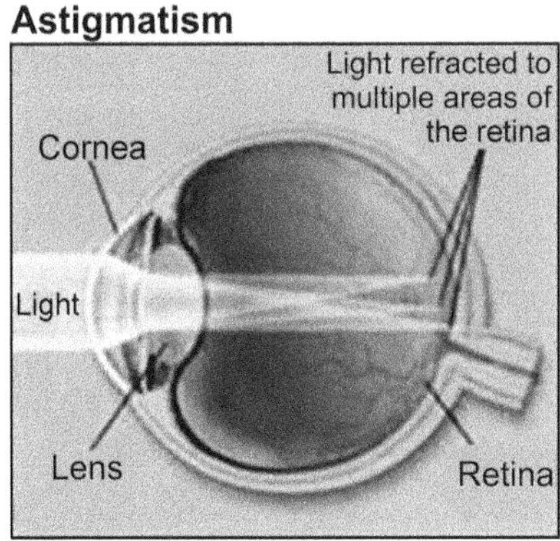

Eye related problems

Cataracts: A cataract is a clouding of the lens, which prevents a clear, sharp image being produced. A cataract forms because the lens is sealed in a capsule and as old cells die they get trapped in the capsule, with time this causes a clouding over of the lens. This clouding results in blurred images.

Age-related macular degeneration (ARMD)

This is a degenerative condition of the macula (the central retina). It is caused by the hardening of the arteries that nourish the retina. This deprives the retinal tissue of the nutrients and oxygen that it needs to function and causes a deterioration in central vision.

Glaucoma: The eye produces a clear fluid (aqueous humour) that fills the space between the cornea and the iris. This fluid filters out through a complex drainage system. It is the balance between the production and drainage of this fluid that determines the eyes intraocular pressure (IOP).Glaucoma is a disease caused by increased IOP usually resulting from a malfunction in the eye's drainage system. Increased IOP can cause irreversible damage to the optic nerve and retinal fibres and if left untreated can result in a permanent loss of vision.

CHAPTER 3

Chemical Hazards

3.1 Introduction to Chemical Hazard

Today, almost every business uses chemicals. Even in the cleanest, most modern office, employees are exposed routinely to inks, toners and adhesives not to mention a wide range of materials used in cleaning and maintenance. Exposure to chemicals in the workplace can cause many different types of harm, ranging from mild irritations to cancer. Managing chemicals and their associated hazards in the workplace will bring real benefits to a business. In addition to improved employee safety and health, cost savings can be achieved by limiting economic losses through effective work practices such as correct storage, handling, use and disposal procedures. Potential harm to the environment will also be reduced.

3.1.1 What are Chemicals?

Most people automatically associate chemicals with scientists in laboratories, but chemicals are also found in many of the products we use at work and at home. While they have a variety of beneficial uses, chemicals can also be extremely harmful if they are misused.

Here are some examples of commonly used household products:

- Cleaning products such as toilet cleaners, disinfectants, mildew remover and chlorine bleach
- Art supplies, such as paint thinner and pottery glazes
- Garage supplies, such as parts degreasers and cleaning solvents
- Office materials, such as photocopier toner

3.1.2 Three Main Chemical States

All chemicals exist in one of three states: solid, liquid or gas.

- A solid has shape and form, whether it's a dust particle or a steel pipe.
- A liquid is a formless fluid. It takes the shape of its container, but doesn't necessarily fill it. Solvents and oils are examples of chemicals in liquid form.

  A gas is a formless substance that expands to occupy all the space of its container. Oxygen and carbon monoxide are examples of chemicals in
- Gaseous form. Gases are usually invisible, but they may be detected in some cases by their taste or smell.

Some chemicals move from one state to another with a change in temperature or pressure. Water is a chemical which is normally a liquid but becomes a solid at temperatures below 0 degrees Celsius.

Knowing the physical states of hazardous chemicals is important factor in understanding their health effects. The physical state of a chemical determines which route it may use to enter the body. For example, a gas may easily enter the body by inhalation, while liquids are more likely to be absorbed through the skin. The fact that chemicals may change their state during work processes that involve changes in temperature and pressure makes it all the more important to take all the possible states of a chemical into account.

3.1.3 Common Chemical Hazards

Specific types of chemicals have been associated with harmful health effects. Common chemical hazards include:

- Skin irritation, disfiguring burns, eye injury or blindness caused bycorrosive chemical products
- Toxic by-products, such as vapours and fumes, caused by mixing incompatible chemicals
- Serious burns from flammable solvents that catch on fire
- Injury from exploding containers, such as spray cans
- Poisoning from accidental swallowing, especially with young children

3.1.4 What does the Law Say?

There are several laws that relate to chemicals in the workplace. Two of the most important laws are:

- The Workplace Hazardous Material Information System (WHMIS)
- The Consumer Products Act and Regulations

WHMIS applies to "controlled products" that meet the government's criteria for a hazardous material. The WHMIS regulation requires labelling, material safety data sheets (MSDS) and training for staff who work with controlled products. WHMIS applies only in the workplace and does not apply to chemical products that you buy for your personal use from a grocery or hardware store. Hazardous substances in the workplace will be labelled with these WHIMIS symbols:

CLASS A

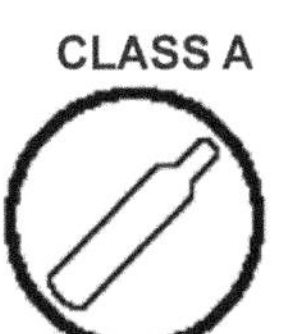

Compressed Gas

CLASS B

Flammable and Combustible Material

CLASS C

Oxidizing Material

CLASS D

1. Materials Causing Immediate and Serious Toxic Effects

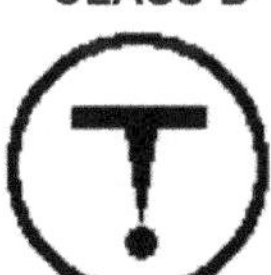

2. Materials Causing Other Toxic Effects

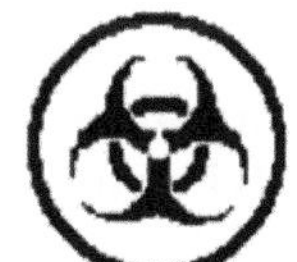

3. Biohazardous Infectious Materials

CLASS E

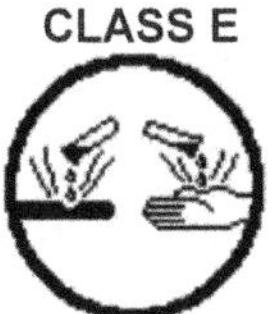

Corrosive Material

CLASS F

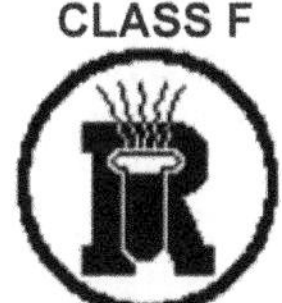

Dangerously Reactive Material

WHMIS Classes and Hazard Symbols

The Consumer Products Act and regulations outlines the requirements for chemical products that you buy for your personal use. Consumer products can be dangerous, so make sure that you read the label on the product and follow the manufacturer's directions for use, clean-up and disposal.

Hazardous consumer products will have these symbols:

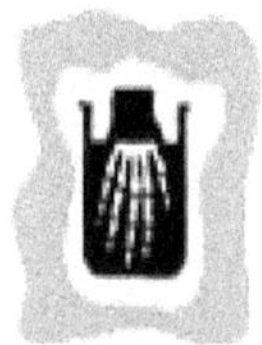
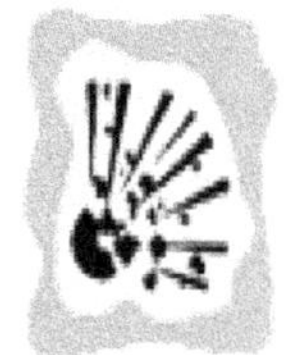
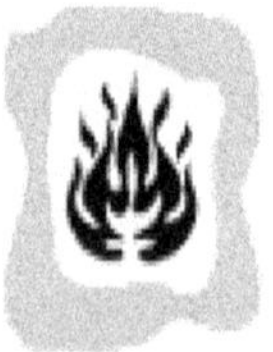
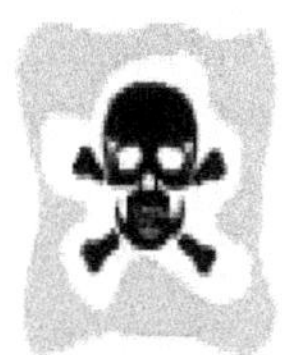

3.1.5 General Tips for Chemical Safety

- Always read the label on the chemical bottle.
- Always follow the directions and precautions listed on the label.
- Never use a chemical if you are unsure what it is or how to protect yourself.
- Always take the time to protect yourself and those working around you.
- Always dispose of a chemical properly. Every municipality has a household hazardous waste drop-off location. For safe disposal of chemical products at work, contact your health and safety representative.

3.1.6 Controlling Chemical Hazards in the Workplace

- Reduce or eliminate the use of hazardous chemicals whenever possible.
- Maintain adequate ventilation systems to reduce concentrations of airborne chemicals.
- Practicing good personal hygiene (e.g. washing hands) and maintaining regular workplace cleaning routines can reduce the amount of a chemical substance that is absorbed by a worker's body. Learn how to avoid carrying hazardous substances home

- Introduce administrative controls to minimize exposure to chemicals (e.g. rotate workers through different jobs or locations, perform maintenance work in off-hours so that accidental release of toxic substances will affect fewer workers).
- Use personal protective equipment and devices.

Maintain equipment in good order to prevent leaks and breakdowns that may release toxic substances.

3.2 Properties of Chemical Dust, Fumes, Smoke, Mist, Vapours and Gases

Dust

Dust include solid particles generated by handling, crushing, grinding, rapid impact, detonation and decrepitating of organic or inorganic materials, such as rock, ore, metal, coal, wood and grain. Dust does not tend to flocculate except under electrostatic forces; it doesn't diffuse in air but settles under the influence of gravity. Dust in the air may or may not have the same composition as its parent material. Dust above 25 mu in size, does not usually remain airborne long enough to pose an inhalation problem to exposed employees, Metals, silica, asbestos etc.

Fumes

Fumes constitute solid particles generated by condensation from the gaseous state, generally after the violation of molten metal's, often accompanied by chemical reaction; fumes coalesce and flocculate. The solid particle that make up fumes are extremely fine, usually less than 0.1 mu, e.g. lead, zinc, cadmium, etc.

Smoke

Smoke carbon or soot particles, less than 0.1 mu in size are caused by the incomplete combustion of carbonaceous materials, such as coal or oil. Smoke generally contains droplets as well as dry particles. The size of the particles contained in tobacco smoke is about 0.25mu.

Mist

Suspended liquid droplets generated by condensation from the gaseous to the liquid state or by breaking up a liquid into dispersed state, such as are known as mist splashing, foaming or atomizing. Mist is formed when a finely divided liquid is suspended in the atmosphere.

Examples of mist are the oil mist produced during cutting and grinding operations, acid mist from electroplating, acid or alkali mists from spraying operations and condensation of water vapour to form fog or rain.

Vapours

Vapours are gaseous forms of substances, which normally exist in solid or liquid state and can return to these states either by increase in pressure or decrease in temperature. Evaporation is the process by which a liquid gets converted into a vapour and mixes with the surrounding atmosphere. Solvents with low boiling points volatilize readily. Examples: Vapours of Trichloroethylene, benzene, xylene, toluene, etc.

Gases

Gases are normally formless fluids that occupy space or an enclosure, and can be changed into liquid or solid into liquid or solid state by the combined effect of increased pressure and decreased temperature. Gases diffuse. For example, welding gases, internal combustion engine exhaust gases, sulphur dioxide, carbon mono oxide, hydrogen sulphide etc.

3.3 Route of Entry to Human System

In order for a chemical to become hazardous to a person's health, it must first contact or enter the body and the chemical must have some biological effect on the body.

There are four major routes:

- Inhalation (breathing)
- Skin contact
- Digestive system (ingestion or eating)
- Injection

Breathing of contaminated air is the most common way that workplace chemicals enter the body. Some chemicals, when contacted, can pass through the skin into the blood stream. Less commonly, workplace chemicals may be swallowed accidentally if food or cigarettes (or hands) are contaminated. For this reason workers should not drink, eat, or smoke in areas where they may be exposed to toxic chemicals.

Injection is the fourth way chemicals may enter the body. While uncommon in most workplaces, it can occur when a sharp object (e.g., needle) punctures the skin and injects a chemical (or virus) directly into the bloodstream.The eyes may also be a route of entry. Usually, however, only very small quantities of chemicals in the workplace enter through the mouth or the eyes.

Regardless of the way the chemical gets into the body, once it is in the body it is distributed to anywhere in the body by the blood stream. In this way, the chemicals can attack and harm organs which are far away from the original point of entry as well as where they entered the body.

What are the parts of the respiratory system that can be affected?

The diagram below shows the parts of the respiratory system. It can divided in two systems - the upper airway passages and the lower airway passages. The upper airway passages includethe nose, nasal passages, mouth and the pharynx down to the vocal cords in the larynx (voice box or "Adam's apple"). The lower airway passages start at the vocal cords, extend down the trachea (windpipe) and continue all the way down to the small air sacs, (alveoli) at the end of every branch of the bronchial tree. The bronchial tree includes the trachea, the bronchus (branches of the trachea going to each lobe of the lung), and bronchioles (branches of the bronchi).

Oxygen in the inhaled breath crosses the alveolar walls to enter the blood within the capillaries. Once oxygen has become attached to the blood inside the veins, it is then distributed throughout the body. Chemical vapors, gases and mists which reach the alveoli in the lungs can also pass into the blood and be distributed around the body.

Sometimes, the concentration of chemicals reaching the alveolar air sacs is lower than in the workplace air. This is because the airways contain a lining of sticky, thick fluid called mucus. Tiny hairs, known as cilia, on the inside of the tubes constantly carry this mucus upwards towards the back of the throat. In some instances, a portion of the gases, vapors and mists may be dissolved in this mucus before they reach the alveolar sacs.

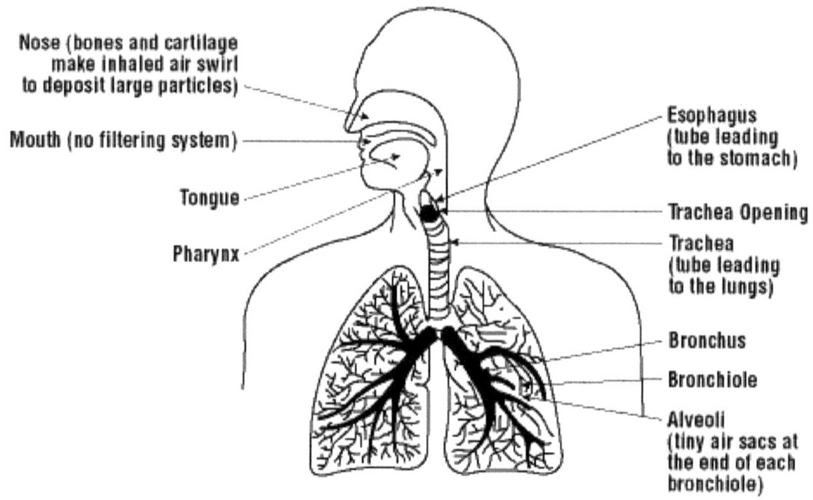

Solid, visible particles found in dusts, fumes and smoke that have escaped the filtering mechanisms of the nose may also be trapped by the mucus. The mucus is wafted by the tiny cilia hairs until it reaches the back of the throat where it is either expelled through the mouth or swallowed and passed to the stomach. In this latter case, the contaminating chemicals will enter the body in the same way as contaminated food or drink. This is dealt with in more detail in the section on the digestive system.

Much smaller particles (so small that they cannot be seen by the eye) may not be stopped by the mucus in the trachea and bronchiole tubes. They travel through the various branches of the airway and eventually reach the alveoli. Solid particles which cannot pass through the thin wall of the air sacs may lodge and stay where they are. Some may dissolve, others may be attacked and destroyed by the scavenger cells of the body's defense system. Others may prove too big or too insoluble to be disposed of in this way and simply stay in the air sacs. Some of these particles, if they are present only in small quantities, do no apparent harm. Other types of dusts may damage the surrounding alveolar walls. The damage may be permanent and may cause scars to form, which eventually interfere with the lung's ability to pass oxygen into the blood stream.

Some acids, caustics or organic chemicals, when inhaled in sizable amounts, can cause serious and irreparable "burn" damage to the mouth, nose, trachea, bronchi and lungs.

Chemical enter body through the skin?

Chemicals which pass through the skin are nearly always in liquid form. Solid chemicals and gases or vapors do not generally pass through the skin unless they are first dissolved in moisture on the skin's surface.

The skin is the second most common route by which occupational chemicals enter the body. It consists essentially of two layers, a thin, outermost layer called the epidermis and a much thicker under layer called the dermis. The epidermis consists of several layers of flat, rather tightly-packed cells which form a barrier against infections, water, and some chemicals. This barrier is the external part of the epidermis. It is called the keratin layer, and is largely responsible for resisting water entry into the body. It can also resist weak acids but is much less effective against organic and some inorganic chemicals. The keratin layer contains fat and fat- like substances which readily absorb chemicals which are solvents for fat, oil, and grease.

Chemicals enter by the skin

Organic and caustic (alkaline) chemicals can soften the keratin cells in the skin and pass through this layer to the dermis, where they are able to enter the veins and hence the blood stream. Areas of the body such as the forearms, which may be particularly hairy, are most easily penetrated by chemicals since they can enter down the small duct containing the hair shaft. Chemicals can also enter through cuts, punctures or scrapes of the skin since these are breaks in the protective layer. Contact with some chemicals such as detergents or organic solvents can cause skin dryness and cracking. There can also be hives, ulcerations or skin flaking. All these conditions weaken the protective layer of the skin and may allow chemicals to enter the body.

Chemicals can vary enormously in the degree to which they penetrate the skin. Some solvents such as trichloroethylene, naphtha and toluene may soften the keratin layer but are not believed to penetrate much further unless there is prolonged skin contact. On the other hand, chemicals such as benzene, carbon tetrachloride, carbon disulfide and methyl alcohol can readily pass through the epidermis and subsequently enter the blood stream. Some chemicals are so corrosive they burn holes in the skin, allowing entry for infection or other chemicals.

In some instances, chemicals may enter by accidental injection through the skin. This may occur in hospital settings or in industrial hole-punching or injection processes. Once in the blood stream, the chemicals can be transported to any site or organ of the body where they may exert their effects.

Chemicals enter digestive system

Chemicals can enter the stomach either by swallowing contaminated mucus which has been expelled from the lungs, or by eating and drinking contaminated food. Food and drink are most frequently contaminated by contact with unwashed hands, gloves or clothing, or by being left exposed in the workplace. Nail-biting and smoking also contribute.

Once inside the mouth, workplace chemicals pass down the esophagus and then into the stomach. Food in the stomach is digested with a strong acid produced by the stomach. A few chemicals, such as alcohol, may pass across the stomach wall and enter the veins and the blood stream here, but most chemicals move from the stomach into a long, twisting tube known as the small intestine. The inside of the small intestine has many hundreds of tiny finger-like projections called villi. The villi have very thin walls and are filled with tiny blood vessels. This allows the digested food to pass from the small intestine across the walls of the villi and enter the veins. The food is then carried around in the blood stream to the parts of the body that need it.

Some workplace chemicals which contaminate food or drink can also pass across the thin walls of the villi and into the blood stream in this manner. Other workplace chemicals, which are not soluble or whose basic units (molecules) are too big to pass across the villi walls, will stay in the gut and pass out through the feces without being absorbed into the blood stream to any extent.

Some acids, caustics and organics may cause severe "burn" damage to the digestive system if ingested in high concentrations.

Chemicals enter through eye

Although eye splashes or eye contamination by workplace chemicals is fairly common, large quantities of chemicals probably do not enter the body this way. Small amounts of chemicals may enter by dissolving in the liquid surrounding the eyes, and larger, but probably not significant amounts, may enter the eyes if they are splashed with chemicals. The eyes are richly supplied with blood vessels and many chemicals can penetrate the outer tissues and pass into the veins. The eye may or may not be damaged during this process, depending on the corrosive nature of the chemical and its ability to penetrate the outer tissues.

3.4 Recognition of Chemical Hazards

The identification of environmental factors and stresses associated with the work and work operations, and understanding of their effects on man and his wellbeing in the workplace and community, is of prime importance.

Recognition, being the first step to be taken in the control of chemical hazards, involves the following:

- Knowledge of the process system
- Entry of worker into the confined spaces for certain operations, which are commonly encountered in an industry, should be recognized as potential hazard operations
- Understanding the health problems inherent in certain workplaces or equipment designs
- Knowledge of toxicity evaluation of all chemicals involved, including initial, intermediate and final products and waste
- Knowledge of the number of persons liable to be exposed and locations of exposure
- Questioning of operators and supervisors and examining work flow sheets

- Spotting hazardous situations before workers are affected
- Matching the symptoms of an ill worker with potential workplace hazards
- Examining compliance status of factories act, with respect to various occupational hazards

3.5 Evaluation

Evaluation is achieved with the aid of quantitative measurement techniques, to measure the magnitude in terms of occupational health hazards factors and stresses that impair human health and well-being.

Evaluation usually requires some form of personal and/or static monitoring to provide a good picture of the level of contamination during the normal work cycle of different workers. There are a variety of monitoring methods that can be used by persons suitably trained and qualified in Industrial Hygiene.

3.5.1 Monitoring Methods

3.5.1.1 Personal monitoring

The concentration of airborne chemicals to which workers are exposed can be determined with the help of sample collecting equipment such as self-contained air samples and air sampling devices worn by workers for determined periods. The selective monitoring of high risk workers, i.e. those who are closet to the source of contaminant generation, is highly recommended. This approach is based on the concept that the probability of significant exposure varies directly with distance from the source. If workers closet to the source are not significantly exposed and probably do not need to be monitored.

Personal monitoring samples should be collected in breathing zone and, if workers are wearing respiratory protective equipment, outside the face piece. These samples represent the actual inhalation exposure of workers who are not wearing respiratory protection and the potential exposure of the workers who are wearing respirators. Personal monitoring may require the use of a variety of sampling media. Unfortunately single workers cannot carry multiple sampling media and if the workers are in team it becomes easier.

3.5.1.2 Environmental monitoring

- Determining the levels of airborne chemical/substances in the working environment can give an indirect estimate of workers exposure and indicate the existence of potential hazards. There are various reasons for establishing environmental monitoring systems the main goals are-
- To provide information about the substances being emitted to the environment, their quantities and sources.
- To determine changes in environmental conditions with time.
- To determine how well the regulatory measures are being met.

The main objective of emission monitoring is to determine the output of ecologically active compounds related to specific processes or parameters. The source from which a pollutant enters the environment may be related to industry, energy conversions, agriculture, or domestic activities. The scale of input to the environment depends on several factors such as kind of processes, size, and number of sources. Environmental monitoring of pollutants at a network of sites in the environment is more difficult to design. The environment receives emissions from a large number of sources and not all the sources are recorded. To obtain a meaningful picture of what is happening demands careful sampling. The system should designed to meet several goals such as it should indicate where and when target exposure is likely to be above the desired levels.

3.5.1.3 Biological monitoring

Biological Monitoring involves measuring the chemical or its metabolite in Biological Agents, such as Blood, Urine, Scalp Hair, Saliva, Nails, Enzymes, Exhaled breath, Body tissues and Body Fluids, and then comparing the levels with the accepted values, as per the standard reference.

The selection of a biological agent for the test mainly depends on the characteristics of the chemicals to be studied. The number of chemicals for which biological monitoring has become available has increased in recent years, but is still small compared to the number of chemicals used in the industry. Biological monitoring has been well recognized in recent years for evaluating the workers exposure to hazardous chemicals. The aim of biological monitoring is to detect hazardous substances in the body before adverse health effect occurs. Where biological monitoring is mandatory employers must ensure that those employees are informed of the requirement to undergo health surveillance before the work commences whereby they may be exposed to that hazardous chemical agent.

When health surveillance involves obtaining biological samples, the procedure must be explained and acceptable to the employees concerned. Workers should be informed that the biological monitoring is voluntary and for their benefit. Employers must maintain an individual health record for each employee who undergoes biological monitoring at his place of work.

3.6 Control of Basic Hazard

Once the hazard is identified and evaluated, residual hazards may be controlled by the application of one of the three principles.

3.6.1 Substitutions

The substitution of hazardous chemicals used in the process with others of lower toxicity.

3.6.2 Containment

The process is engineered or modified so that hazardous products are completely contained and disposed of safely.

3.6.3 Reduction

The level of workers exposure should be reduced to a safe level by engineering control methods (isolation/enclosure, ventilation) and improving housekeeping, personal hygiene and maintenance.

3.6.4 Administrative control

Administrative controls limit workers exposures by scheduling shorter times in contaminant areas or by implementing other rules

- Scheduling maintenance and other high exposure operations for times when few workers are present.

- Using job-rotation schedules that limit the amount of time an individual worker is exposed to a substance.
- Using a work-rest schedule that limits the length of time a workers is exposure to a hazard.

3.6.5 Employer must Ensure that

- Workers who work with or near controlled products are properly trained.
- Supplier or work site labels are present on containers of controlled products.
- Current and correct Material Safety Data Sheets (MSDS) are readily available for all controlled products.
- Procedures and training are developed in consultation with the joint occupational Health and Safety Committee if there is one.

3.7 Concepts of the Dose-Response Relationship

It quantitatively defines the role of the dose of a chemical in evoking a biological response. In the absence of chemical no response is seen. As chemical is introduced into the system the response is initiated at the threshold dose and increases in intensity as the dose is raised. Ultimately a dose is reached beyond which no further increase in response is observed. The dose-response relationship can be demonstrated for interactions of chemicals with biological receptors leading to physiological responses, therapeutic effects of drugs, or for toxic, lethal, teratogenicity, mutagenic or carcinogenic effects of chemicals. The data from these studies can be expressed as dose-response curves which can take the form of linear plots or a variety of reciprocal or logarithmic transformations.

Two types of dose-response relationships are observed. The first is the incremental change in response of a single system or individual as the dose is increased. The second is the distribution of responses in a population of individuals given different doses of the agent. The former are frequently used for the determination of the mechanism of interaction between the chemical and the biological system. The latter describe the response of a population of individuals and can also be used to determine multimodal responses indicative of genetic variations.

The dose-response relationship is of key importance when attempting to define allowable exposure of humans to chemicals in the workplace, consumer products or the environment. Usually initial studies are done in animals and, where possible, they are compared with data derived from recorded human exposure. The reliability of extrapolations from these data is compromised by the inherent inaccuracy of the data observed in the high and, more importantly, the low dose regions of the dose-response curves since these usually demonstrate the fewest responses. It is essential that we develop new approaches to understanding responses to low doses of chemicals if we are to define safe limits of exposure with accuracy.

3.8 Threshhold Limit Value

American Conference of governmental industrial hygienists (ACGIH) which publishes these values (TLVs) annually, defines airborne concentrations to which, it is believed, most workers may be repeatedly exposed without adverse effects.

If includes concepts like:

(a) **Time weighted Average Concentrations (TWACs):** Applicable to repeated exposure of workers for an 8 hour duration per day, during a normal Working week without adverse effects.

(b) **Short Term Exposure limits (STELs)**: Applicable to workers with an exposure for a period up to 15 minutes, with no more than four such exposures per day (during 8 hours shifts), and at least 60 minutes between them.

(c) **Ceiling values (CV):** exposure should never exceed any of the above periods.

Threshold Limit value (TLVs) are derived from experience and experimental work and are supported by published material of the ACGIH, stating the sources used to define each value and the underlying objective, whether it is protection of health or comfort and amenity.

In India, TLVs, published by ACGIH, are adopted as threshold limit value.

3.9 Air Sampling Strategies

1. When conducting hygiene monitoring or measurements, the following sampling strategies shall as far as possible be followed:-

   (a) The atmosphere of any workplace in which toxic airborne contaminants are given off shall be monitored at sufficient intervals.

   (b) Occupations with the highest expected exposure shall be monitored first. Representative subjects shall be selected for sampling.

   (c) All monitoring shall represent the personal exposure unless otherwise specified. The monitoring device should be attached as close as possible to the worker's breathing zone. Note the periods when exposure may be high due to specific activities or process cycles. Change the sample collection medium when conditions show signs of overloading due to excessive airborne contaminants.

   (d) If area monitoring is conducted, the monitoring device or sampling medium shall be positioned at about 1.2 to 1.8 meter (3 to 4 feet) from the floor. Make sure that the sample collection medium is not in direct contact with, or placed too close to any settled dust or spilled chemical.

   (e) Samples representing a full-shift exposure shall be collected for evaluating or assessing the time weighted average (TWA) concentration.

   (f) Before conducting the air monitoring, the air monitoring service provider shall obtain from the factory occupier or his representative the information on the work process to be monitored. The information shall be recorded in Part C of the Hygiene Air Monitoring Report -Information on Work Process.

   (g) A minimum of 6 hours of sampling is required to evaluate exposure over a full 8-hour shift, or 8 hours of sampling for a full 12-hour shift. However, this is only applicable to work processes with small concentration variations. Otherwise, a full shift (8 or 12 hours) sampling is required.

   If the worker is exposed to contaminants for less than 6 hours, a partial-period sampling could be conducted covering the period of exposure. In this case, the period, which was not sampled, could be assumed to have zero exposure. [An example of the calculation of TWA8hr concentration is in appendix 1].

2. All sampling and monitoring shall be carried out in accordance with the recommended procedures. Ensure that all active monitoring devices are calibrated. Before use, check the batteries of the devices for charge and the expiring date of the sampling medium. In addition, make sure that the following are carried out: -
   (a) Sample collection medium (membrane filter) for monitoring of total particulate shall be desiccated for at least 24 hours prior to weighing. If vacuum desiccators are used, desiccation of filter can be reduced to 30 minutes.
   (b) Sorbent tube used for monitoring of gases or vapours shall be positioned vertically to avoid "Channeling" (i.e. the adsorbent shifts and forms a channel within the tube) during sample collection. After sampling, the sorbent tube shall be capped at both ends and stored at <4□C prior to analysis in order to prevent sample loss.
3. All equipment and instruments used for sampling shall be calibrated in accordance with standard calibration methods before and after sampling. The persons carrying out the air monitoring must ensure that the sampling equipment used is reliable and accurately calibrated.
4. The person carrying out the monitoring shall as far as possible remain at the workplace until all the samples are collected. He should ensure that the monitoring devices are not tampered with. He should also check the flow rate of the monitoring devices after the first 15-30 minutes and at intervals of about two hours thereafter.
5. The sample size should be at least 3 to 5 samples per job-classification/group, or from 25% to 50% of those in the group for groups of 10 or more.
6. The frequency of air monitoring depends on the exposure level: -

   < 10 % of the PEL: * No air monitoring is required.

   10 – 50% of the PEL: At least once a year.

   > 50 – 100% of the PEL: At least once every six months

3.10 Bio Chemical Action of Toxic Substances

Toxic materials can cause serious health effects in an exposed individual. The degree of hazard associated with any toxic material is related to the exact material you are exposed to, concentration of the material, the route into the body and the amount absorbed by the body (the dose). Individual susceptibility of the user also plays a role.

The health effects may occur immediately or the effects may be delayed. Health effects that occur immediately after a single exposure are called acute effects. In other cases, health effects will not occur until some point after the exposure. This is called a chronic effect. A chronic effect may occur hours, days, months or even years after exposure. Generally, acute effects are caused by a single, relatively high exposure. Chronic effects tend to occur over a longer period of time and involve lower exposures (e.g., exposure to a smaller amount over time). Some toxic materials can have both acute and chronic health effects.

It is important to remember that toxic materials can have other hazards associated with it. For example, a toxic material may also be corrosive and flammable. Always read the Material Safety Data Sheet and labels to be sure you understand what is in the product and how to work with it safely. If you do not understand the instructions, or if you are not sure, check with your supervisor.

Biochemical responses of animals to environmental chemicals (biochemical biomarkers) can give measures of exposure, and sometimes also toxic effect. They are particularly valuable where they can be used to measure the toxic effects of chemicals in the field, employing non-destructive sampling methods. Measurements of exposure are useful in the case of non-persistent chemicals (e.g. organ phosphorus, carbamate, or pyrethroid insecticides) which are difficult or impossible to detect by chemical analysis. They can also be useful to provide an integrated measure of the level of exposure to a group of related chemicals. Biochemical biomarkers are likely to provide a measure of toxic effect, where they are based upon a molecular mechanism which underlies toxicity. A widely-used biochemical biomarker is cholinesterase depression, which may involve destructive sampling (brain acetyl cholinesterase) or non-destructive sampling (serum butyrylcholinesterase). For genotoxic chemicals, techniques which measure DNA damage (e.g. detection of DNA adducts) provide a powerful tool in measuring environmental effects. The detection of biochemical changes caused by anticoagulant rodenticides (e.g. abnormal levels of clotting proteins in blood) provides another example of this approach. In general, the development of simple, sensitive, and specific assays that are 'user-friendly' would open the way for much wider use of biochemical biomarkers in environmental monitoring.

3.11 Biological Sampling and Analysis

Chemical sampling and analysis is used by occupational health and safety professionals to assess workplace contaminants and associated worker exposures. The validity of an assessment is based, in part, on the procedures used for sample collection and analysis, and data interpretation. Sampling and analysis hazards are addressed in specific standards for the general industry.

Effective and efficient sampling strategies require planning and foresight to ensure the most productive and thorough evaluation of contaminants in the workplace. The following references provide information about chemical sampling.

3.11.1 Survey Protocol

Prior to conducting chemical sampling a survey protocol should be developed. This protocol serves as a guide in performing the survey. The amount of detail necessary will depend on the purpose of the survey and to whom the results will be submitted. At a minimum, the protocol should include the following:

- Purpose of the survey. Why the survey being conducted and what is the desired outcome? Background information such as previous surveys, operational or equipment changes should be referenced.
- Where to sample? This identifies expected exposure sites. It is based on where chemicals are stored, transported, and used at the site, and what ventilation and airflow patterns exist.
- What to sample? This is based on available information. What are the potential chemical hazards?

- Who to sample? This is based on knowledge of the potential exposure sites and the various job requirements at the site. What job classifications or specific individuals should be considered for monitoring? Workers with the greatest potential for exposure must be included.
- How many samples should be collected? Consider the number of exposure sites, job classifications, and potential chemical hazards. How many samples are necessary to assess the various exposure hazards?
- How will the samples be collected and analysed? After determining the potential hazards, what published methods are available, and which ones will provide the most meaningful data. Is there a potential for other chemical hazards in the area and should methods be considered which may provide screening information?

3.11.2 Sampling Methods

3.11.2.1 Direct reading

Direct reading instruments provide an excellent mechanism to monitor potential exposures. They allow significant amounts of data to be collected and the workers exposure profile during operations to be determined. They, also, provide qualitative data relative to worker exposures. However, they may not provide the necessary specificity, detection limit, or precision for compliance monitoring or exposure assessment.

3.11.2.2 Bulk samples

Bulk samples may be collected and shipped to the laboratory as an aid in assessing sources of contamination. In order to prevent contamination of personal samples, they should be kept separate from the personal samples when transporting and packaged in separate containers when shipping.

Analysis Procedure

The hazard analysis procedure has been broken down into the five following activities. Applying them in a logical sequential manner will help to avoid any omissions. Once these five activities have been completed we will have an extensive list of realistic potential hazards:

1. Review incoming material

2. Evaluate processing operations for hazards
3. Observe actual operating practices
4. Take measurements
5. Analyse
6. The measurements

3.12 Work Environment Monitoring

Employers are required by the Health and Safety in Employment Act to provide their employees with a healthy and safe working environment. For many, this will involve monitoring both the environment in the workplace, and the employees themselves for levels of harmful chemicals.

A wide range of monitoring methods can be used. These include:

1. Sampling pumps, with appropriate tubes and filters
2. Colour tubes
3. Passive sampling badges
4. Direct reading instruments, for real-time readout of results
5. Data logging instruments for collecting data over time
6. Biological monitoring

CHAPTER 4

Personal Protective Equipment

Introduction

PPE (i.e. Personal protective equipment) is briefly explained in this record of assignment. It consists of Definition of PPE, why it is needed, methods for selection of PPE, Different types of PPE, respective usage of devices, proper selection of requirement, maintenance of PPE, Testing procedures to selection and standards for devices of PPE.

The main objective of this record is to occupational safety and workplace hazards regarding Construction Industry is elaborated. And the Complete scenario of PPE for Industries also included for working safely.

What is personal protective equipment?

Personal protective equipment, commonly referred to as "PPE", is equipment worn to minimize exposure to serious workplace injuries and illnesses. These injuries and illnesses may result from contact with chemical, radiological, physical, electrical, mechanical, or other workplace hazards. Personal protective equipment may include items such as gloves, safety glasses and shoes, earplugs or muffs, hard hats, respirators, or coveralls, vests and full body suits.

4.1 Need for PPE

Getting your workers to take care of themselves can sometimes be the hardest part of supervising them. After a while you may give up on the particularly stubborn ones...But for leaders in safety this can never be an option! While you are legally responsible for the safety of your employees while they are in your workplace, your employees need to know how much responsibility they have on their shoulders in terms of working safely; both for themselves and for their colleagues.

At the end of the day, no matter how many safety precautions we take and how many measure we implement to reduce and eliminate safety hazards, people still get hurt. This is reality. But one thing that can absolutely be done as a minimum to try to control risks is using personal protective equipment (PPE) properly.

Now, it is certainly your job as a safety leader to train people in what they need to be using, how it needs to be used, when it needs to be used, and to supervise the use of the PPE, but at the end of the day, it is in the employee's hands to actually do it. And it will be their injury if this doesn't happen. It is so essential to teach your employees the basics so that they understand the aim of what they might consider to be a lot of red tape.

So while we have our procedures and policies and records and slogans, it is so important to have the physical measures in place that can make a real difference in preventing injuries and illnesses in your workplace. Making the workplace safe includes providing instructions, procedures, training and supervision to encourage people to work safely and responsibly. Even where engineering controls and safe systems of work have been applied, some hazards might remain.

These include injuries to:

- the lungs, e.g., from breathing in contaminated air
- the head and feet, e.g., from falling materials
- the eyes, e.g., from flying particles or splashes of corrosive liquids
- the skin, e.g., from contact with corrosive materials
- the body, e.g., from extremes of heat or cold.

PPE is needed in these cases to reduce the risk.

4.2 Method for Selection of PPE

Selection of PPE

First of all select the job, process or procedure you are going to assess. Survey the worksite and identify the hazards the worker will be exposed to while doing the work. Use copy of the certificate of Hazard Assessment Form or Work sheet or one of your own to list the identified hazards.

For each of the identified hazards review the discussion of control and PPE options in the hazard control and PPE section remember, control methods should be implemented first. If PPE must be used, list the PPE that will be used for each hazard identified on your form or work sheet. After the assessment and selection, employees required to use PPE must be trained. All in the following must be covered.

- Tell them which PPE they must use and when to use it
- Discuss the limitation of the PPE
- Show them how to put it on, take it off and adjust it
- Show the users how to inspect and maintain the PPE
- Make sure you have covered everything in the instructions that come with the PPE and the warning labels on the equipment itself
- Make sure the PPE fits well
- Tell them how to get the required PPE
- Have them demonstrate that they understand the training

Assure that current employees have received the required PPE training. Establish a mechanism for assuring all new employees are trained before they are required to use the PPE.

The training must be repeated if:

- The workers don't understand how to use the equipment
- The workers are using the equipment improperly, or
- The job changes so the PPE requirements change

There are some examples for selection of PPE in different types of hazards:

(i) **Biohazards (Germs):** We should use splash goggles, respirators, gloves, surgical masks, lab coats, aprons, and sleeves for biohazards.

(ii) **Bright light (welding, lasers, and glass blowing)**: For these type of hazards we should use glasses, goggles, face shield PPEs.

(iii) **Chemicals**: During chemicals situation we can used these types of PPE –respirators, gloves, shoe covers, chemical resistant clothing, vapour proof or splash goggles.

(iv) **Dust:** For dust we should use dust goggles, respirators.

(v) **Falling objects:** In this condition we should use hard hats, steel toe shoes, metatarsal guards.

(vi) **Fall from a height**: Safety harness, fall arrest system, hard hats these PPE should use in falls from a height.

(vii) **Noise:** In noisy condition we should use hearing protector's ear plugs and ear muffs to prevent from noise hazards.

4.3 Non-Respiratory PPE (Pesonal Protective Equipment)

There are mainly two types of PPE:-

(i) Respiratory and

(ii) Non respiratory

RESPIRATORY PPEs are used when air is contaminated with toxic gases and breathing in the atmosphere is not safe in these conditions this type of PPEs are used. And NON RESPIRATORY PPEs are used in every condition where hazards are not possible to eliminate, substitute, controlling by engineering and controlling by administration, then lastly we use PPE (respiratory and non-respiratory).

Non respiratory PPEs are listed below which are:

A. Helmet

B. Safety goggles

C. Ear plugs/Ear muffs

D. Gloves

E. Safety shoes and safety boots

F. Face shield and

G. Welding shield, etc

4.3.1 PPE for Head

Head is a very important part of human body, injury to head causes serious effects on human body & also may cause death. So head protection is very much important while working in an industry.

Potential Head Hazards present at workplaces:

- Impact

- Falling or flying objects
- Hitting head to hard objects
- Injuries include neck sprains, concussions, and skull fractures
- Electric Shock
- Exposureto live electric wires
- Injuries include electrical shocks and burns
- Drips
- Toxic liquids such as acids, caustics, and molten metals can irritate and burn the head/scalp.

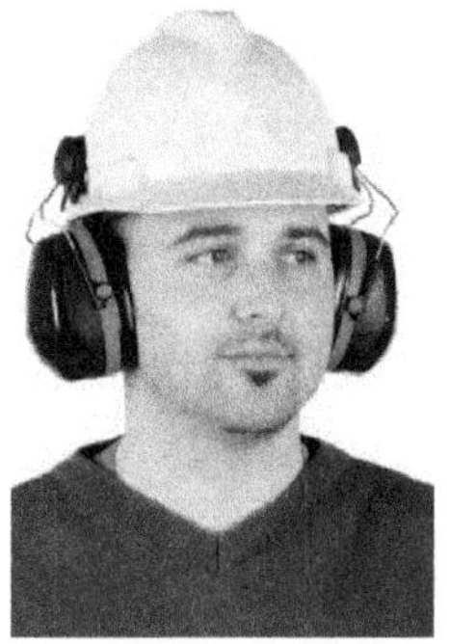

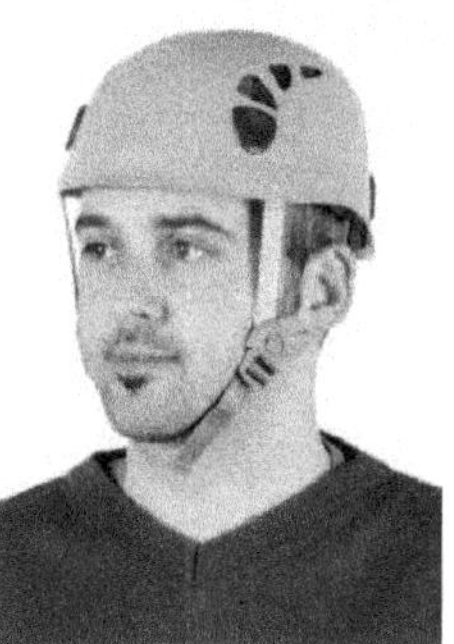

Industrial safety helmet (With fitted ear defenders) Climbing helmet

Mostly Hard hats are used as PPE for head protection as is has following properties

- A rigid shell that resists and deflects blows to the head
- A suspension system inside the hat that acts as a shock absorber
- Some hats serve as an insulator against electrical shocks

Types of PPE's for Head Protection-

Class A Hard Hats:

- Protect from falling objects.
- Protect from electrical shocks up to 2,200 volts.

Class B Hard Hats:

- Protect from falling objects.
- Protect from electrical shocks up to 20,000 volts.

Class C Hard Hats:

- Protect from falling objects.
- Bump Caps

Bump caps are made from lightweight plastic and are designed to protect you from bumping your head on protruding objects.

Proper use and care of hard hat

- Always wear your hard hat while you are working in areas where there are potential head hazards
- Adjust the suspension inside your hard hat so that the hat sits comfortably, but securely on your head
- Inspect the shell of your hard hat for cracks, gouges, and dents. Inspect the suspension system for frayed or broken straps. If you're hard hat needs to be repaired, have it repaired immediately or ask your employer for a new one
- Place plastic (non-metal) reflective tape on hat if working at night
- Never paint, scratch or drill "air holes" in your hard hat
- Never carry personal belongings such as cigarettes, lighters, or pens in your hard hat
- Clean your hard hat at least once a month by soaking it in a solution of mild soap and hot water for 5-10 minutes
- Because sunlight and heat can damage the suspension of your hat, always store your hat in a clean, dry, and cool location

4.3.2 PPE for EARS

Hearing protection should only be used where risks to hearing remain despite the implementation of other measures to control the noise, or while those other measures are being developed or put in place.

Generally, the louder the noise, the shorter the exposure time before hearing protection is required. For instance, employees may be exposed to a noise level of 90 dB for 8 hours per day (unless they experience a Standard Threshold Shift) before hearing protection is required. On the other hand, if the noise level reaches 115 dB hearing protection is required if the anticipated exposure exceeds 15 minutes.

Some types of hearing protection include:

Single-use earplugs

They are made of waxed cotton, foam, silicone rubber or fiberglass wool. They are self-forming and, when properly inserted, they work as well as most molded earplugs.

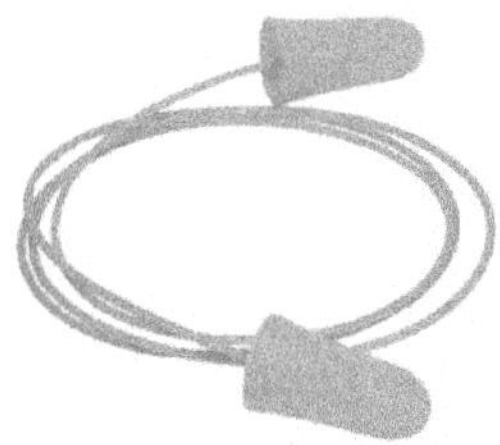

Pre-formed or molded earplugs

Must be individually fitted by a professional and can be disposable or reusable. Reusable plugs should be cleaned after each use.

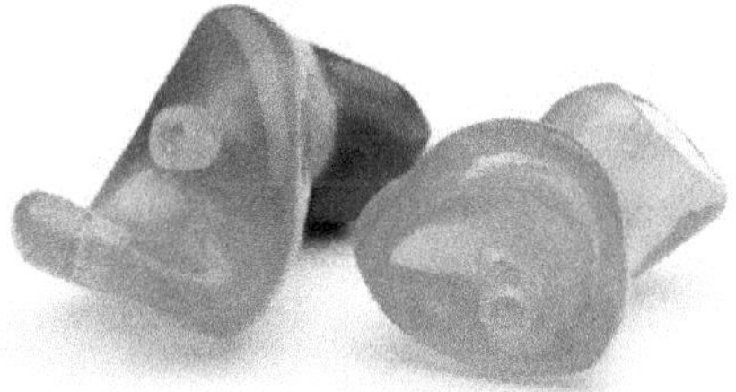

Earmuffs

Require a perfect seal around the ear. Glasses, facial hair, long hair or facial movements such as chewing may reduce the protective value of earmuffs.

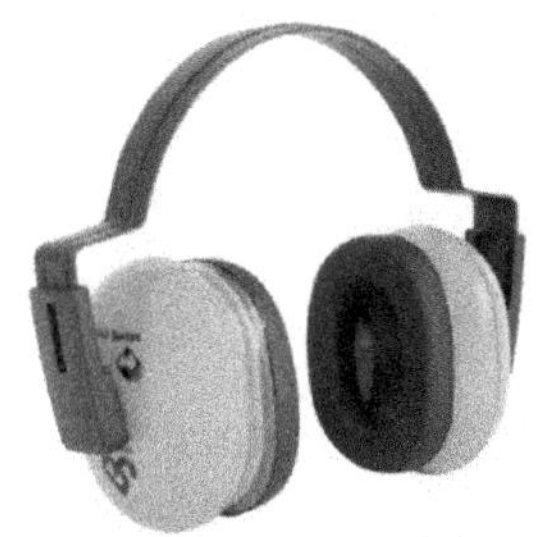

4.3.3 PPE for Eyes

Thousands of people are blinded each year from work related eye injuries. Types of eye & face hazards-

Impact

Small particles of matter can enter eyes and damage them. Operations such as grinding, chiseling, sanding, hammering, and spraying can create small airborne particles.

Heat

Welding, working near boilers, furnaces etc.

Chemicals

Toxic chemicals in the form of gases, vapours, and liquids can damage your eyes. Always read the appropriate MSDS before working with any hazardous material.Always check with your supervisor or safety manager to learn the type of eye or face protection you will need to use in order to work safely

Dust

Material handling, construction and demolition.

Light and/or Radiation

Welding, metal cutting, and working around furnaces etc. expose the workers to heat, glare, ultraviolet, and infrared radiation.

Types of Eye and Face Personal Protective Equipment

Safety Glasses

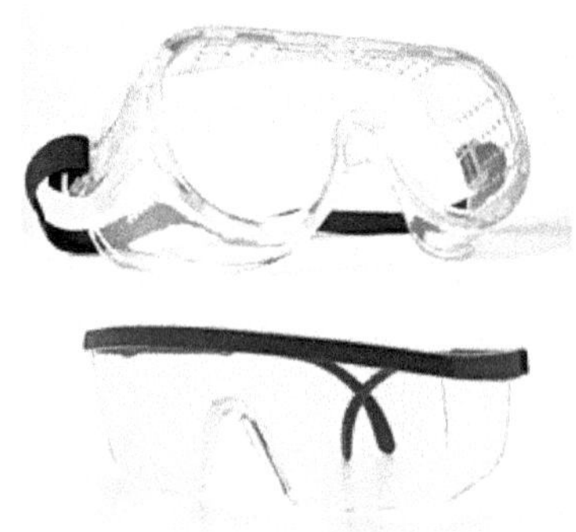

Much stronger and more resistant to impact and heat than regular glasses. Equipped with side shields that give protection

from hazards that may not be directly in front. Safety glasses should be z-87 approved to meet she regulations. Should fit comfortable on face through all job tasks. Ensure that glasses are not too big or too tight.

Limitations

Does not seal around eyes, could allow small droplets to come in contact with eyes

Goggles

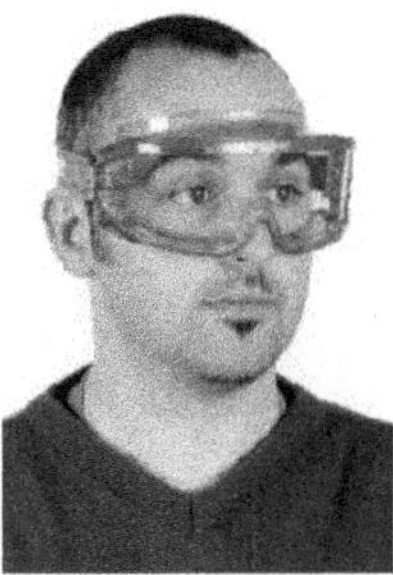

Surround the eye area; they give you more protection in situations where you might encounter splashing liquids, fumes, vapours, powders, dusts, and mists

Must indicate that they are chemical splash goggles to be worn for that purpose

Limitations

Uncomfortable to wear with other head gear like helmet, ear muffs or respirator.

Face Shields

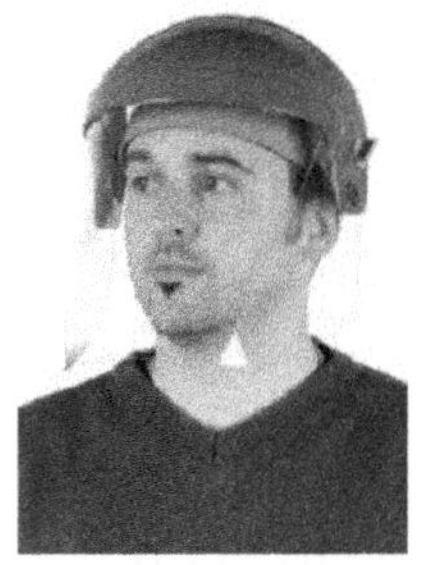

Full face protection Used around operations which expose you to molten metal, chemical splashes, or flying particles. Can be used simultaneously as a hard hat.

Limitations

Are not considered eye protection, will need to wear goggles or glasses underneath. Can fog up if working in poorly ventilated area.

Welding Helmets

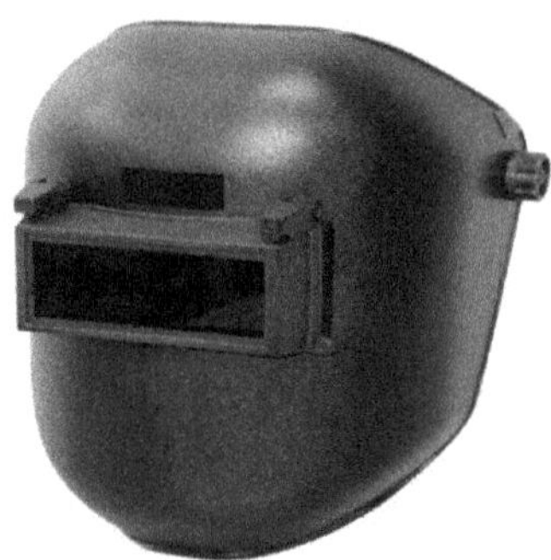

Provide both face and eye protection. Use special absorptive lenses that filter the intense light and radiant energy that is produced during welding operations.

Limitations

- Heavy and hot, fog up.
- Must wear safety glasses or goggles underneath helmet.
- Absorptive Lenses
- Additional protection if you worker has to work where there is bright light or glare.

Limitations

- Must be used in conjunction with safety glasses or goggles.
- Care of Eye Protection Equipment-
- Clean the eye protection equipment with mild soap and water.
- Abrasive soaps, rough paper, or cloth towels should never be used.
- Keep PPE in good working condition.
- If damaged, replace it as soon as possible.

- Store eye protection equipment in a sanitary, cool, dry area away from moisture & dust.
- Read the manufacturer's directions and warnings before using any eye protection equipment.

4.3.4 Hand Protection

If a workplace hazard assessment reveals that employees face potential injury to hands and arms that cannot be eliminated through engineering and work practice controls, employers must ensure that employees wear appropriate protection. Potential hazards include skin absorption of harmful substances, chemical or thermal burns, electrical dangers, bruises, abrasions, cuts, punctures, fractures and amputations.

Protective equipment includes gloves, finger guards and arm coverings or elbow-length gloves. Employers should explore all possible engineering and work practice controls to eliminate hazards and use PPE to provide additional protection against hazards that cannot be completely eliminated through other means. For example, machine guards may eliminate a hazard. Installing a barrier to prevent workers from placing their hands at the point of contact between a tables saw blade and the item being cut is another method.

Types of Protective Gloves

There are many types of gloves available today to protect against a wide variety of hazards. The nature of the hazard and the operation involved will affect the selection of gloves. The variety of potential occupational hand injuries makes selecting the right pair of gloves challenging. It is essential that employees use gloves specifically designed for the hazards and tasks found in their workplace because gloves designed for one function may not protect against a different function even though they may appear to be an appropriate protective device. The following are examples of some factors that may influence the selection of protective gloves for a workplace.

- Type of chemicals handled.
- Nature of contact(total immersion, splash, etc.).
- Duration of contact.
- Area requiring protection (hand only, forearm, arm).

- Grip requirements (dry, wet, oily).
- Thermal protection.
- Size and comfort.
- Abrasion/resistance requirements. Gloves made from a wide variety of materials are designed for many types of workplace hazards.
- In general, gloves fall into **four groups**
- Gloves made of leather, canvas or metal mesh;
- Fabric and coated fabric gloves;
- Chemical- and liquid-resistant gloves;
- Insulating rubber gloves

Leather, Canvas or Metal Mesh Gloves

Sturdy gloves made from metal mesh, leather or canvas provide protection against cuts and burns. Leather or canvass gloves also protect against sustained heat

- Leather gloves protect against sparks, moderate heat, blows, chips and rough objects.
- Aluminized gloves provide reflective and insulating protection against heat and require an insert made of synthetic materials to protect against heat and cold.
- Aramid fibre gloves protect against heat and cold, are cut- and abrasive-resistant and wear well.
- Synthetic gloves of various materials offer protection against heat and cold, are cut- and abrasive-resistant and may withstand some diluted acids. These materials do not stand up against alkalis and solvents.

Fabric and Coated Fabric Gloves

Fabric and coated fabric gloves are made of cotton or other fabric to provide varying degrees of protection.

- Fabric gloves protect against dirt, slivers, chafing and abrasions. They do not provide sufficient protection for use with rough, sharp or heavy materials. Adding a plastic coating will strengthen some fabric gloves.
- Coated fabric gloves are normally made from cotton flannel with napping on one side. By coating the unmapped side with plastic, fabric gloves are transformed into general-

purpose hand protection offering slip-resistant qualities. These gloves are used for tasks ranging from handling bricks and wire to chemical laboratory containers. When selecting gloves to protect against chemical exposure hazards, always check with the manufacturer or review the manufacturer's product literature to determine the gloves' effectiveness against specific workplace chemicals and conditions.

Chemical and Liquid-Resistant Gloves

Chemical-resistant gloves are made with different kinds of rubber: natural, butyl, neoprene, nitrile and fluorocarbon (Viton); or various kinds of plastic: polyvinyl chloride (PVC), polyvinyl alcohol and polyethylene. These materials can be blended or laminated for 24 better performance. As a general rule, the thicker the glove material, the greater the chemical resistance but thick gloves may impair grip and dexterity, having a negative impact on safety. Some examples of chemical-resistant gloves include:

- **Butyl gloves** are made of a synthetic rubber and protect against a wide variety of chemicals, such as peroxide, rocket fuels, highly corrosive acids (nitric acid, sulphuric acid, hydrofluoric acid and red-fuming nitric acid), strong bases, alcohols, aldehydes, ketones, esters and nitro compounds. Butyl gloves also resist oxidation, ozone corrosion and abrasion, and remain flexible at low temperatures. Butyl rubber does not perform well with aliphatic and aromatic hydrocarbons and halogenated solvents.
- **Natural (latex) rubber gloves** are comfortable to wear, which makes them a popular general-purpose glove. They feature outstanding tensile strength, elasticity and temperature resistance. In addition to resisting abrasions caused by grinding and polishing, these gloves protect workers' hands from most water solutions of acids, alkalis, salts and ketones. Latex gloves have caused allergic reactions in some individuals and may not be appropriate for all employees. Hypoallergenic gloves, glove liners and powerless gloves are possible alternatives for workers who are allergic to latex gloves.

- **Neoprene** gloves are made of synthetic rubber and offer good pliability, finger dexterity, and high density and tear resistance. They protect against hydraulic fluids, gasoline, alcohols, organic acids and alkalis. They generally have chemical and wear resistance properties superior to those made of natural rubber.
- **Nitrile** gloves are made of a copolymer and provide protection from chlorinated solvents such as trichloroethylene and perchloroethylene. Although intended for jobs requiring dexterity and sensitivity, nitrile gloves stand up to heavy use even after prolonged exposure to substances that cause other gloves to deteriorate. They offer protection when working with oils, greases, acids, caustics and alcohols but are generally not recommended for use with strong oxidizing agents, aromatic solvents, ketones and acetates.

Different types of hand gloves

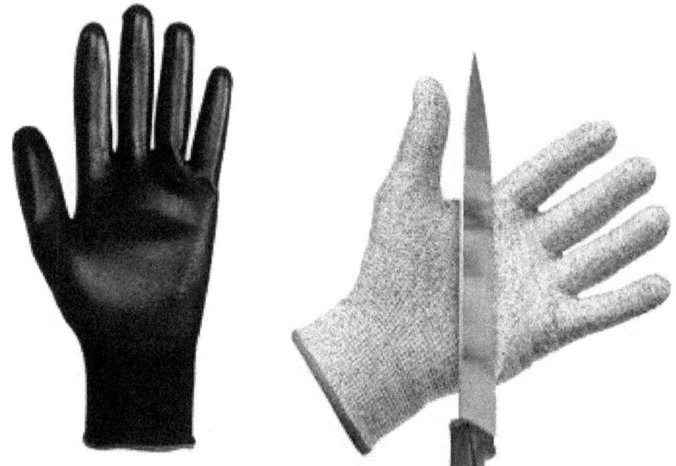

Hand Gloves

4.3.5 Foot Protection

In designing strategies to protect foot injury, one has to remember the fundamental principle of occupational health and safety: those occupational hazards should be eliminated at the source. The role of personal protective equipment is to minimize exposure to specific occupational hazards, not to eliminate them.

Protective footwear does not guarantee total protection for workers exposed to foot hazards, the required protection is protective footwear certified by the CSA Group.

All working footwear, for both men and women, whether it is safety wear or not, should provide comfort without compromising protective value. In addition, protective footwear should conform to CSA Standard CAN/CSA-Z195-14 or appropriate standard for your jurisdiction.

A steel toe cap should cover the whole length of the toes from tips to beyond the natural bend of the foot. A soft pad covering the edge of the toecap increases comfort. If the toecap cuts into the foot, either the size or style of the footwear is incorrect. Soles come in a variety of thicknesses and materials. They need to be chosen according to the hazards and type(s) of flooring in the workplace. Uppers of protective footwear come in a variety of materials. Selection should take into account the hazards, and individual characteristics of the worker's foot.

A steel midsole which protects the foot against penetration by sharp objects should be flexible enough to allow the foot to bend. No one type of non-slip footwear can prevent the wearer from slipping on every surface type.

Steps for taking foot care

- Feet are subject to a great variety of skin and toenail disorders. Workers can avoid many of them by following simple rules of foot care:
- Wash feet daily with soap, rinse thoroughly and dry, especially between the toes.
- Trim toenails straight across and not too short. Do not cut into the corners.
- Wear clean socks or stockings and change them daily.
- Some feet sweat more than others and are more prone to athlete's foot. Again, following a few simple guidelines may help:
- Select shoes made of leather or canvas – not synthetic materials.
- Keep several pairs of shoes on hand and rotate shoes daily to allow them to air out.

- For some workers, non-coloured woollen or cotton socks may be recommended since dyes may cause or aggravate skin allergies.
- Use foot powder.
- If problems persist, see a doctor or health care specialist.
- In cases of persisting ingrown toenails, calluses, corns, fungal infection and more serious conditions such as flat feet and arthritis, see a doctor and follow the doctor's advice.

Foot protection against cold weather can be resolved by

- Insulating the legs by wearing thermal undergarments
- Wearing insulating overshoes over work footwear
- Wearing insulating muffs around the ankles and over the top of the footwear

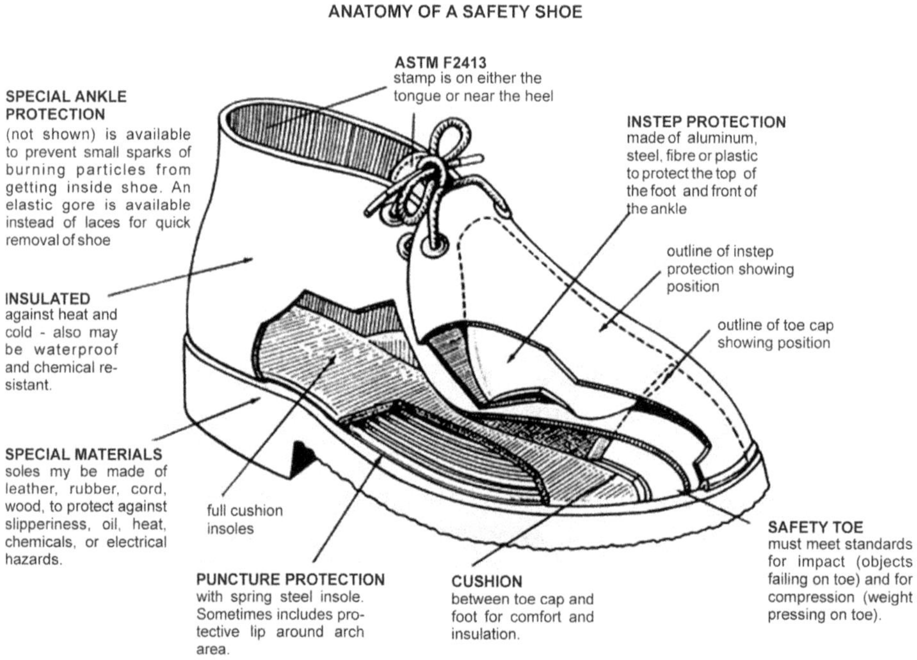

Different Types of Safety Shoes

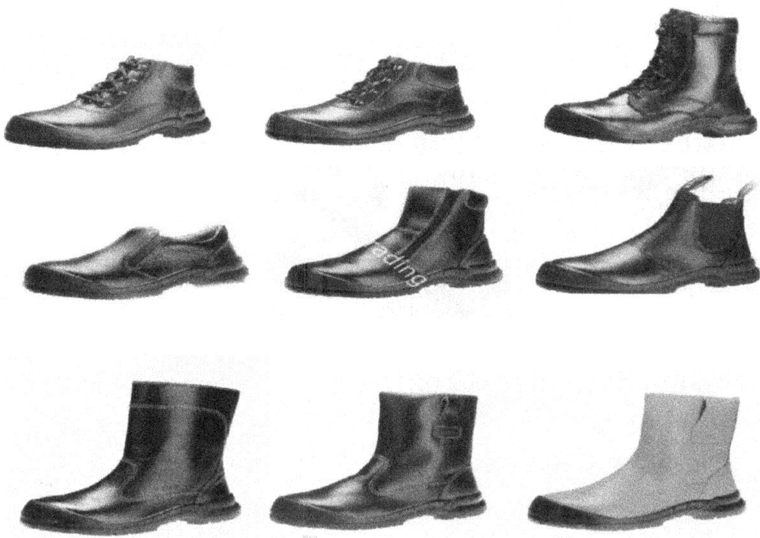

4.3.6 Body Protection

Safe Operating Procedure

This safe operating procedure provides information on the selection and use of outer garments, such as suits, chaps, vests, sleeves, coats, etc., to protect the body from injury. Specialized operations, such as PPE to protect against electrical shock/arc flash, are beyond the scope of this safe operating procedure.

Body Hazards

- Exposure to sharp knives or power cutting tools (i.e., chainsaw, etc.);
- Exposure to temperature extremes (i.e., intense summer heat or winter cold, working in walk-in freezers/coolers, etc.);
- Contact with intense heat, including molten metals and other hot materials (e.g., steam, sparks, etc.);
- Contact with pesticides and other chemicals;
- Working with radioactive materials;
- Contact with infectious materials, including blood and body fluids;

- Contact with rough or abrasive surfaces;
- Working around motorized vehicles, operating bicycles, and other situations where there is a need to enhance a person's visibility.

Materials of Construction

Many different materials of construction are available for various protective body garments.

- Paper-like fibre used for disposable suits provide protection against dust and small splashes.
- Treated wool and cotton adapts well to changing temperatures, is comfortable, fire-resistant and protects against dust, abrasions, and rough and irritating surfaces.
- Duck is a closely woven cotton fabric that protects against cuts and bruises when handling heavy, sharp, or rough materials.
- Leather is often used to protect against dry heat and flames.
- Rubber, rubberized fabrics, neoprene and plastics protect against certain chemical and physical hazards. When chemical or physical hazards are present, check with the clothing manufacturer to ensure that the material selected will

Specialized Body Protection

- High Visibility. Body protection garments are available to enhance a person's visibility (e.g., workers in construction zones, traffic controllers, etc.).
- Welding aprons, sleeves, bibs, and coats are available to protect against hot splashes from molten metal's, Safety in Welding, Cutting, and Allied Processes.

However, this standard does not incorporate specific garment test protocols like it does for welding helmets and protective eyewear. Rather, it states: "Clothing shall provide sufficient coverage, and be made of suitable materials, to minimize skin burns caused by sparks, spatter, or radiation." Heavier materials such as woollen clothing or heavy cotton are preferable to lighter materials because they are more difficult to ignite. Cotton clothing, if used for protection, should be chemically treated to reduce its combustibility.

Chainsaws, In the United States, the primary performance standard for chainsaw is to select a manufacturer that adheres to this standard or an equivalent international consensus standard.

Cut-resistance, Clothing to help protect against cuts can be made from a variety of materials. Most often, this type of clothing is not associated with any particular performance standard. Thus, selection is largely based on good judgment. In some cases, such as typical kitchen operations, sufficient protection may be afforded by

A heavy apron. However, in a meat-packing-like operation Kevlar or stainless steel mesh may be more appropriate. The key is to select a product that is well matched to the risk.

General Guidance on Proper Use

Regardless of the type of protective garment used:

- Protective clothing should be carefully inspected before each use, it must fit each worker properly, and it must function properly and for the purpose for which it is intended.
- The general PPE use considerations and information provided for protective gloves also apply to garments used for body protection. See SOP, Personal Protective Equipment – Hand Protection.
- PPE should be stored in a well-ventilated, clean, and dry environment, away from

Direct sunlight and contaminants. Sometimes, a manufacture will specify storage of certain PPE in sealed bags

- Users of any type of PPE must read and adhere to the manufacturer's use and maintenance instructions. These instructions should be kept in a manner that they can be easily referenced from time-to-time.
- Do not reuse disposable/single use PPE.
- Decontaminate reusable PPE immediately after use and in accordance with manufacturer's instructions.
- All PPE should be inspected prior to each use to verify its integrity.
- Compromised PPE should be removed from service.

- Refrain from wearing items that could compromise the integrity of the PPE. For example, sharp tools carried in pockets could penetrate protective coveralls.

Different Types of Body Protection Equipment's

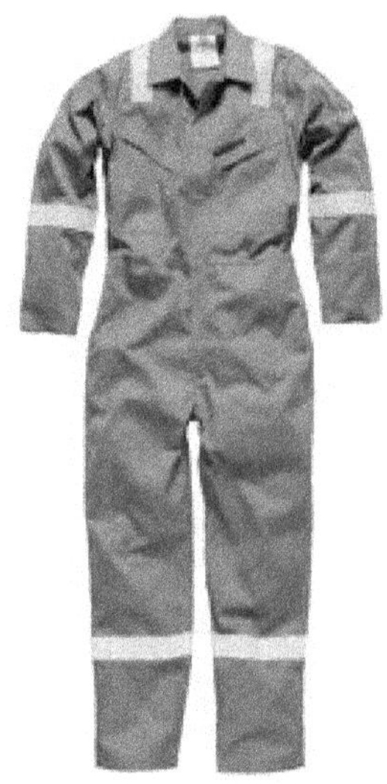

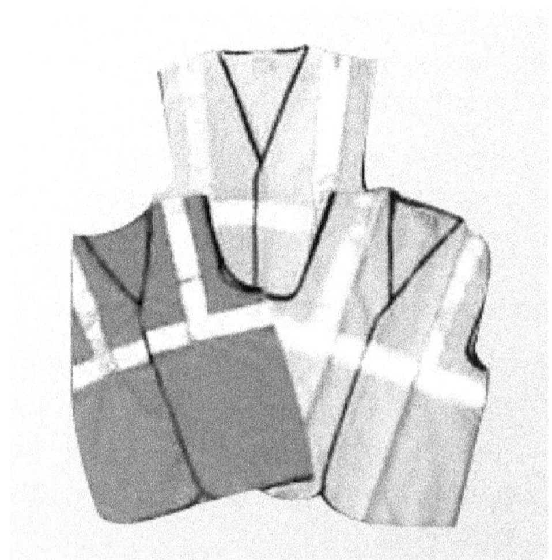

4.4 Respiratory PPE

A respirator is a protective device that covers the nose and mouth or the entire face or head to guard the wearer against hazardous atmospheres.

Respirators may be

Tight-fitting

That is, half masks, which cover the mouth and nose and full face pieces that cover the face from the hairline to below the chin; or

Loose-fitting

Such as hoods or helmets that cover the head completely. In addition, there are two major classes of respirators: Air-purifying, which remove contaminants from the air; and Atmosphere-supplying, which provide clean, breathable air from an uncontaminated source. As a general rule, atmosphere-supplying respirators are used for more hazardous exposures.

When employees must work in environments with insufficient oxygen or where harmful dusts, fogs, smokes, mists, fumes, gases, vapours, or sprays are present, they need respirators. These health hazards may cause cancer, other diseases where toxic substances are present in the workplace and engineering controls are inadequate to reduce or eliminate them, respirators are necessary. Some atmosphere-supplying respirators can also be used to protect against oxygen-deficient atmospheres. Increased breathing rates, accelerated heartbeat, and impaired thinking or coordination occur more quickly in an oxygen-deficient or other hazardous atmosphere. Even a momentary loss of coordination can be devastating if it occurs while a worker is performing a potentially dangerous activity such as climbing, working at heights etc. Employees need to wear respirators whenever engineering and work practice control measures are not adequate to prevent atmospheric contamination at the worksite. Strategies for preventing atmospheric contamination may include enclosing or confining the contaminant-producing operation, exhausting the contaminant, or substituting with less toxic materials. Respirators have their limitations and are not a substitute for effective engineering and work practice controls. When it is not possible to use these controls to reduce airborne contaminants below their occupational exposure levels, such as during certain maintenance and repair operations, emergencies, or when engineering controls are being installed, respirator use may be the best or only way to reduce worker exposure. In other cases, where work practices and engineering controls alone cannot reduce exposure levels to below the occupational exposure level.

OSHA's respirator standard requires employers to establish and maintain an effective respiratory protection program when employees must wear respirators to protect against workplace hazards. Different hazards require different respirators, and employees are responsible for wearing the appropriate respirator and complying with the respiratory protection program.

The standard contains requirements for program administration, worksite-specific procedures, respirator selection, employee training, fit testing, medical evaluation, and respirator use, cleaning, maintenance, and repair. Employees must use respirators while effective engineering controls, if they are feasible, are being installed. If engineering controls are not feasible, employers must provide respirators and employees must wear them when necessary to protect their health.

The employee's equipment must be properly selected, used, and maintained for a particular work environment and contaminant. In addition, employers must train employees in all aspects of the respiratory protection program.

4.4.1 Classification of Respirators

The purpose of a respirator is to prevent the inhalation of harmful airborne substances and/or an oxygen-deficient atmosphere. Functionally, a respirator is designed as an enclosure that covers the nose and mouth or the entire face or head. Respirators are of two general "fit" types, tight-fitting and loose-fitting. The tight-fitting respirator is designed to form a seal with the face of the wearer. It is available in three types: quarter mask, half mask, and full face piece. The quarter mask covers the nose and mouth, where the lower sealing surface rests between the chin and the mouth. The half mask covers the nose and mouth and fits under the chin. The full face piece covers the entire face from below the chin to the hairline.

The loose-fitting respirator has a respiratory inlet covering that is designed to form a partial seal with the face. These include loose-fitting face pieces, as well as hoods, helmets, blouses, or full suits, all of which cover the head completely. The best known loose-fitting respirator is the supplied air hood used by the abrasive blaster. The hood covers the head, neck, and upper torso, and usually includes a neck cuff. Air is delivered by a compressor through a hose leading into the hood. Because the hood is not tight-fitting, it is important that sufficient air is provided to maintain a slight positive-pressure inside the hood relative to the environment immediately outside the hood. In this way, an outward flow of air from the respirator will prevent contaminants from entering the hood.

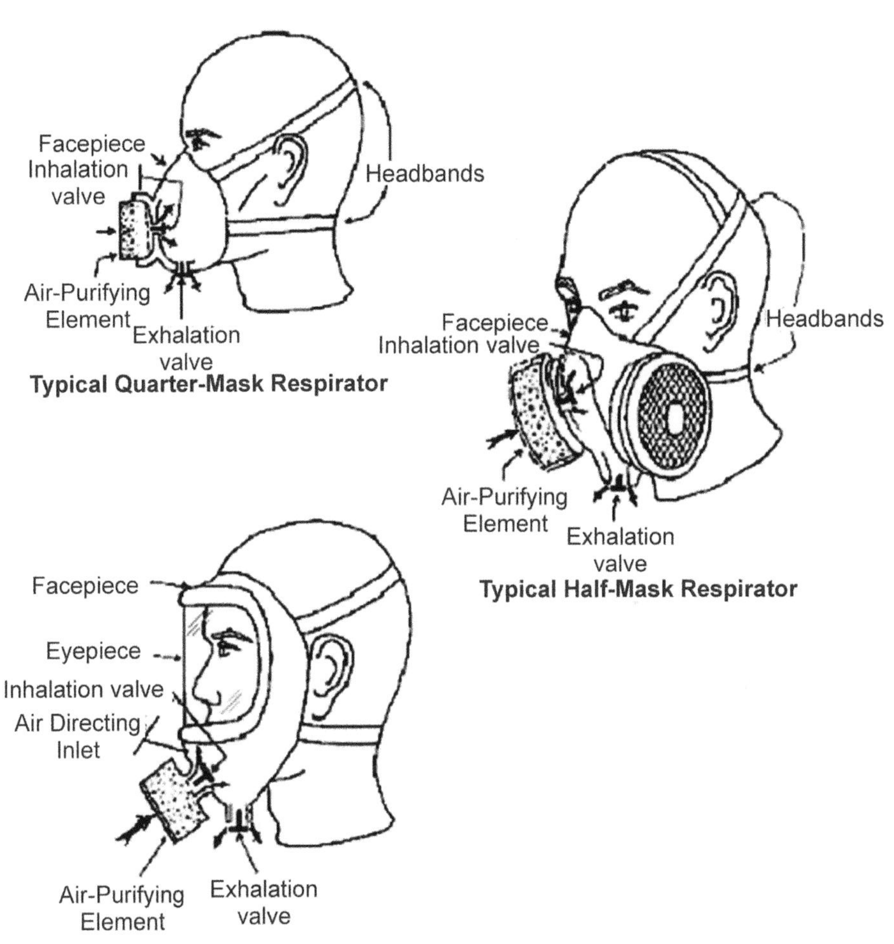

Tight-Fitting Respirators

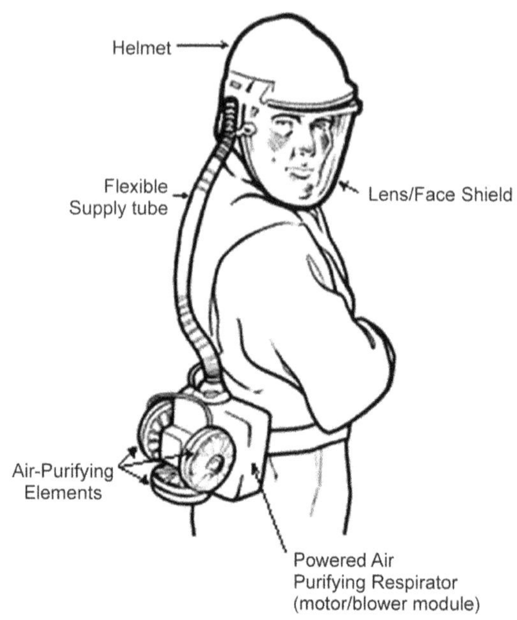

Loose-Fitting Facepiece

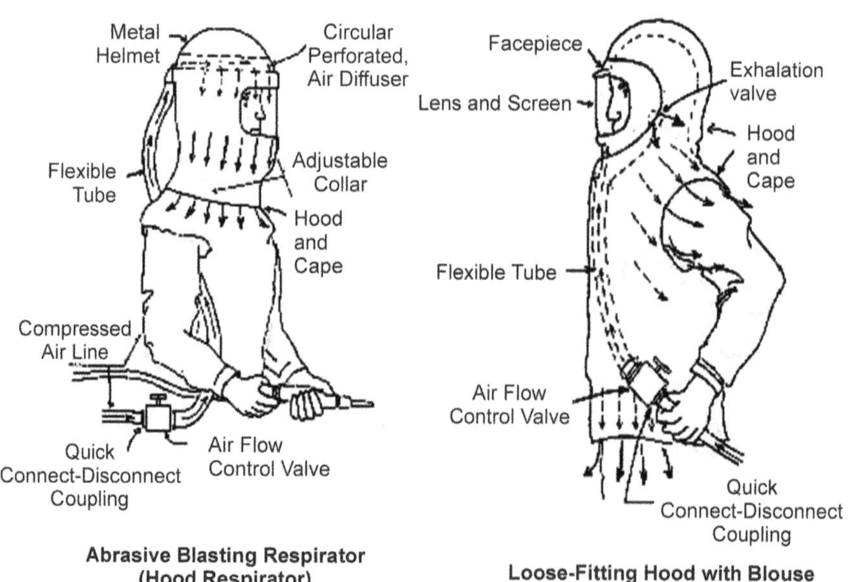

Abrasive Blasting Respirator (Hood Respirator)

Loose-Fitting Hood with Blouse

Loose-Fitting Respirators

Airborne (or Respiratory) Hazards

May result from either an oxygen deficient atmosphere or breathing air contaminated with toxic particles, vapours, gases, fumes or mists. The proper selection and use of a respirator depend upon an initial determination of the concentration of the hazard or hazards present in the workplace, or the presence of an oxygen deficient atmosphere.

Airborne hazards generally fall into the following basic categories

Dusts

Particles those are formed or generated from solid organic or inorganic materials by reducing their size through mechanical processes such as crushing, grinding, drilling, abrading, or blasting.

Fumes

Particles formed when a volatilized solid, such as a metal, condenses in cool air. This physical change is often accompanied by a chemical reaction, such as oxidation. Examples are lead oxide fumes from smelting, and iron oxide fumes from arc-welding. A fume can also be formed when a material such as magnesium metal is burned or when welding or gas cutting is done on galvanized metal.

Mists

A mist is formed when a finely divided liquid is suspended in the air. These suspended liquid droplets can be generated by condensation from the gaseous to the liquid state or by breaking up a liquid into a dispersed state, such as by splashing, foaming, or atomizing. Examples are the oil mist produced during cutting and grinding operations, acid mists from electroplating, acid or alkali mists from pickling operations, paint spray mist from spraying operations, and the condensation of water vapor to form a fog or rain.

Gases

Gases are formless fluids that occupy the space or enclosure and which can be changed to the liquid or solid state only by the combined effect of increased pressure and decreased temperature. Examples are welding gases such as acetylene, nitrogen, helium and argon; and carbon monoxide generated from the operation of internal combustion engines. Another example is hydrogen sulfide, which is formed wherever there is decomposition of materials containing sulfur under reducing conditions.

Vapours

Vapours are the gaseous form of substances that are normally in the solid or liquid state at room temperature and pressure. They are formed by evaporation from a liquid or solid, and can be found where parts cleaning and painting takes place and where solvents are used.

Smoke

Smoke consists of carbon or soot particles resulting from the incomplete combustion of carbonaceous materials such as coal or oil. Smoke generally contains droplets as well as dry particles.

Oxygen deficiency

An oxygen deficient atmosphere has oxygen content below 19.5% by volume. Oxygen deficiency may occur in confined spaces, which include, but are not limited to, storage tanks, process vessels, towers, drums, tank cars, bins, sewers, septic tanks, underground utility tunnels, manholes, and pits.

Respirator Classifications

Respirators provide protection either by removing contaminants from the air before they are inhaled or by supplying an independent source of reparable air.

There are two major classifications of respirators:

Air purifying respirators (devices that remove contaminants from the air); and **Atmosphere-supplying respirators** (those devices that provide clean breathing air from an uncontaminated source).Each class of respirator may have tight-fitting and loose-fitting face pieces. An important aspect of respirator operation and classification is the air pressure within the face piece. When the air pressure within the face piece is negative during inhalation with respect to the ambient air pressure, the respirator is termed a negative-pressure respirator. When the pressure is normally positive with respect to ambient air pressure throughout the breathing cycle, the respirator is termed a positive-pressure respirator. The concept of negative and positive pressure operation is important when considering potential contaminant leakage into the respirator.

Air Purifying Respirators

Are grouped into three general types: particulate removing, vapor and gas removing, and combination. Elements that remove particulates are called filters, while vapor and gas removing elements are called either chemical cartridges or canisters. Filters and canisters/cartridges are the functional portion of air-purifying respirators, and they can generally be removed and replaced once their effective life has expired. The exception would be filtering face piece respirators (commonly referred to as "disposable respirators," "dust masks," or "single-use respirators"), which cannot be cleaned, disinfected, or resupplied with an unused filter after use.

Particulate-removing respirators are designed to reduce inhaled concentrations of nuisance dusts, fumes, mists, toxic dusts, radon daughters, asbestos-containing dusts or fibres, or any combination of these substances, by filtering most of the contaminants from the inhaled air before they enter the breathing zone of the worker. They may have single-use or replaceable filters. These respirators may be non-powered or powered air-purifying. A powered air-purifying respirator (PAPR) uses a blower to force the ambient atmosphere through air purifying elements to the inlet covering.

Vapor- and gas-removing respirators are designed with sorbent elements (canisters or cartridges) that adsorb and/or absorb the vapors or gases from the contaminated air before they can enter the breathing zone of the worker. Combination cartridges and canisters are available to protect against particulates, as well as vapors and gases.

Atmosphere Supplying Respirators

Are respirators that provide air from a source independent of the surrounding atmosphere instead of removing contaminants from the atmosphere? These respirators are classified by the method that is used to supply air and the way in which the air supply is regulated. Basically, these methods are: self-contained breathing apparatus (air or oxygen is carried in a tank on the worker's back, similar to SCUBA gear); supplied-air respirators (compressed air from a stationary source is supplied through a high-pressure hose connected to the respirator); and combination self-contained and supplied-air respirators.

Limitations of Respirator

Not all workers can wear respirators. Individuals with impaired lung function, due to asthma or emphysema for example, may be physically unable to wear a respirator. Individuals who cannot get a good face piece fit, including those individuals whose beards or sideburns interfere with the face piece seal, will be unable to wear tight-fitting respirators. An adequate fit is required for a respirator to be effective. In addition to these problems, respirators may also be associated with communication problems, vision problems, fatigue, and reduced work efficiency.

In principle, respirators usually are capable of providing adequate protection. However, problems associated with selection, fit, and use often render them less effective in actual application; these problems prevent the assurance of consistent and reliable protection, regardless of the theoretical capabilities of the respirator. Occupational safety and health experts have spent considerable effort over the years developing fit-testing procedures and methods of measuring respirator effectiveness, thereby improving protection for those employees required to wear them.

4.4.2 Selection of Respiratory PPE

Respirator selection requires correctly matching the respirator with the hazard, the degree of hazard, and the user. The respirator selected must be adequate to effectively reduce the exposure of the respirator user under all conditions of use, including reasonably foreseeable emergency situations. Proper respirator selection involves choosing a device that fully protects the worker from the respiratory hazards to which he or she may be exposed and permits the worker to perform the job with the least amount of physical burden.

Selection Factors

Many factors must be considered carefully in respirator selection. In choosing the appropriate respirator, one must consider the nature and extent of the hazard, work requirements and conditions, and the characteristics and limitations of the respirators available. The following categories of information must be taken into account:

- Nature of the hazard, and the physical and chemical properties of the air contaminant
- Concentrations of contaminants
- Relevant permissible exposure limit or other occupational exposure limit
- Nature of the work operation or process
- Time period the respirator is worn
- Work activities and physical/psychological stress
- Fit testing; and
- Physical characteristics, functional capabilities and limitations of respirators

Nature of the hazard, and the physical and chemical properties of the air contaminant. The nature of the hazard, whether it is in the form of a gas, dust, organic vapor, fume, mist, oxygen deficiency or any combination of hazards, needs to be taken into account. The physical and chemical properties of the contaminant that affect respirator selection, and the selection of respirator components such as cartridges, canisters, and filters must also be considered. Physical properties include such factors as particle size for dusts, and vapor pressure for gases and vapors. Chemical properties of the air contaminant that affect breakthrough times, and the ability of the filter material to remove, adsorb, or absorb the contaminant must also be considered. Concentrations of contaminants. Sampling and analysis of the workplace air determines what degree of exposure is occurring, and thus what degree of protection is required. Where such sampling and analysis have been done, the results are to be used as a point of comparison with the occupational exposure level, i.e., to determine how much the concentration must be lowered by the respirator to reduce employee exposure to a safe level.

The relevant permissible exposure limit or other occupational exposure limit. Respirators selected must be capable of protecting against overexposure by reducing and maintaining exposure to or below the relevant exposure limit. In addition to the OSHA limits, employers should refer to the ACGIH (American Conference of Governmental Industrial Hygienists) recommended

Threshold Limit Values (TLV's), the NIOSH (National Institute for Occupational Safety and Health) Recommended Exposure Limits (REL's), or other occupational exposure limits.

Nature of the work operation or process. The type of job operation, the equipment or tools that will be used, and any motion or travel the job requires can influence the type of respirator selected, particularly when supplied-air respirators, which require a connection to a clean air source, are used.

Time period respirator is worn. The employer must also consider the period of time during which the respirator will be used by employees during a work shift. Breakthrough times for different chemicals can vary greatly, and are dependent on the concentrations of contaminants in the workplace air, patterns of respirator use, and environmental factors including temperature and humidity. A respirator that provides adequate protection for one chemical may be inadequate for another chemical with a different breakthrough time. In addition, employees wearing respirators for longer periods of time may need respirators that impose the minimum possible physical burden. Work activities and stress. The work activities of employees while wearing respirators are also a factor. Heavy work that is physically draining may affect an employee's capability of wearing certain types of respirators. Temperature and humidity conditions in the workplace may also affect the physical/psychological stress level associated with wearing a respirator, as well as the effectiveness of respirator filters and cartridges. These types of factors must be assessed in selecting the appropriate equipment for a particular work situation.

Fit testing

Some employees may be unable to achieve an adequate fit with certain respirator models or a particular type of respirator -- such as half-mask air-purifying respirators so an alternative respirator model with an adequate fit or other type of respirator that provides adequate protection must be used. Therefore, it is necessary for employers to provide a sufficient number of respirator models and sizes from which employees can choose an acceptable respirator that fits correctly. Physical characteristics, functional capabilities, and limitations of respirators. The last category of information to be considered when selecting respiratory protection is the physical characteristics, functional capabilities, and limitations of the respiratory protection equipment itself. Respirators selected must not impair the worker's vision, hearing, communication, and physical movement necessary to perform jobs safely. For example, airline respirators should not be used by mobile employees around moving machinery to avoid entanglement of the respirator in the equipment.

Selection

Once the above factors have been taken into account, the employer must select a NIOSH-certified respirator. Where NIOSH has not specifically certified any respirator for use against the particular contaminant present in the workplace, the employer must select a NIOSH-certified respirator that has no limitation prohibiting its use for that contaminant. The respirator must be appropriate for the contaminant's physical form and chemical properties and the conditions under which it will be used. All respirators must be chosen and used according to the limitations of the NIOSH certification, which appears on the NIOSH certification label. Until such time as OSHA addresses the issue of assigned protection factors (APF's), employers may rely on APF's published by NIOSH and ANSI. Where there are conflicts between the NIOSH and ANSI APF's, the employer should apply the more protective APF.

Warning System

When an air-purifying respirator is selected for protection against gases and vapors, a system must be in effect that will reliably warn respirator wearers of contaminant breakthrough. These systems are: a respirator equipped with an end-of-service life indicator (ESLI) certified by NIOSH for the contaminant, or an established and enforced cartridge/canister change schedule that is based on objective information or data that will ensure that canisters and cartridges are changed before the end of their service life.

Atmospheres Requiring Highest Level of Protection

For atmospheres that are immediately dangerous to life and health (IDLH), the highest level of respiratory protection and reliability is required. These atmospheres, by definition, are the most dangerous environments in which respirators are used. In these atmospheres, there is no tolerance for respiratory failure.

Consequently, only the following respirators must be provided and used: full-face piece pressure demand self-contained breathing apparatus (SCBA) certified for a minimum service life of thirty minutes, or a combination full-face piece pressure demand supplied-air respirator (SAR) with an auxiliary self-contained air supply.

4.4.3 Instructions and Trainings in the Use

Where PPE is provided employees must be informed of the risks against which they are being protected by the PPE. Employees must also be provided with suitable information, instruction and training (including training in the use, care or maintenance of PPE) to enable them to make proper and effective use of any PPE provided for their protection.PPE users must be trained as regards the wearing, proper use and any limitations of PPE. Managers and supervisors should also be aware of the reasons for providing PPE, its proper use and, in particular, the level of protection afforded. Training, both theoretical and practical, should also cover persons involved in the selection, maintenance, repair and testing of PPE. After selecting suitable PPE, the employer should inform the employees what PPE has to be used for a particular risk, why to use it, when to use it and how to use it. Such messages are most appropriately conveyed to the employees through a component of the PPE programme: information, instruction and training.

This component of the PPE programme deals with many factors related to human behavior. To make the component successful, the employer should, after consulting their employees, develop an effective plan for the following:

(a) Establishing in-house safety rules to provide instructions regarding use of PPE;

(b) Providing access of necessary safety and health information to the employees, e.g. chemical hazards in the workplace and safety precautions; safety information about PPE

(c) Establishing appropriate training policy for his employees;

(d) Reinforcing information, instruction and training by

  (i) observation, supervision and inspection of employees in performing their jobs;

  (ii) Promotional activities to encourage the use of PPE;

(iii) Use of signs and posters at various working zones that require the use of PPE.

(e) Establishing commending and reprimanding mechanism for the PPE programme;

Information and instruction should cover:

- The risk(s) present and why the PPE is needed
- The operation (including demonstration), performance and limitations of the equipment
- Use and storage (including how to put it on, how to adjust and remove it)
- Any testing requirements before use
- Any user maintenance that can be carried out (e.g. hygiene/cleaning procedures)
- Factors that can affect the performance of the equipment (e.g. working conditions, personal factors, defects and damage)]
- How to recognise defects in PPE, and arrangements for reporting them
- Where to obtain replacement PPE
- The way in which the PPE controls the risks and its limitations
- Why the PPE is appropriate
- The way to use the PPE to ensure that it is effective and, when appropriate, test it

Where necessary, train and instruct workers to put on and remove contaminated clothing without contaminating themselves. The extent of the training required will depend on the type of equipment, how frequently it is used and the needs of the staff being trained. Anyone involved in a supervisory role must also have adequate training and instruction relating to PPE in order for them to have the necessary skills to spot potential bad practices, defects or incorrect use of equipment by staff. Training records should be kept wherever more than very simple instruction is required.

Information and instruction can be provided to the employees by following means

(a) Documentation in the form of safety manual, work procedures and emergency

Procedures is the primary means and the documents should be located in prominent

Locations in the workplace accessible by the employees.

(b) Other means such as notices, placards, posters, video show should also be used as appropriate in arousing the safety awareness of employees on using PPE.

Training of employees

Training helps employees in acquiring the necessary attitude, knowledge and skills in order to be competent in using PPE for handling and use of chemicals. Comprehensive training programme should be provided to everyone who is involved in the use or maintenance of PPE. Users should be trained in the proper use of PPE, how to correctly fit and wear it, and what the limitations are. Managers and supervisors should also be aware of why PPE is being used and how it is used properly. Employees involved in maintaining, repairing and testing the equipment should also be trained. Training should include elements of theory as well as practice in using the equipment, and should be carried out in accordance with the recommendations and instructions supplied by the PPE manufacturer.

Theoretical training should include

(a) Explanation of the risks present and why PPE is needed;

(b) The operation, performance and limitations of the equipment;

(c) Instruction on the selection, use and storage of PPE related to the intended use;

(d) Written operating procedures such as permits to work involving PPE should be Explained;

(e) Factors which can affect the protection provided by the PPE such as compatibility

With other protective equipment, personal factors, working conditions, inadequate Fitting, as well as defect, damage and wear; and

(f) Recognising defects in PPE and arrangements for repair or replacement.

Practical training should include

(a) Practice in putting on, wearing and removing the equipment;

(b) Practice and instruction in inspection and, where appropriate, testing of the PPE Before use

(c) Practice and instruction in the maintenance which can be done by the user, such as

Cleaning and the replacement of certain components; and

(d) Instruction in the safe storage of equipment. Personal protective equipment training needs can be separated into induction, more specific job training and ongoing training.

Induction Training

General information about personal protective equipment should form an integral part of a workplace's induction training program for its new workers. This training should cover arrangements for the provision, use, storage and maintenance of personal protective equipment as well as emergency procedures in the case of special risks, for example chemical spills or fires.

Specific Job Training

Training for specific jobs involves providing information about the risks associated with the job as identified through the risk management process. Specific job training should also provide instruction in the use of personal protective equipment required for the job, including:

- Recognition of the need for personal protective equipment;
- Basic design principles of the equipment;
- Correct use and wearing of personal protective equipment, as specified by the manufacturer or
- Supplier and/or in the relevant Australian Standard;
- Comfort and fit requirements;
- Application and effectiveness of a selected item;
- Limitations in use, including any limit on the duration for which it can be safely used;
- Maintenance and replacement procedures, as specified by the manufacturer or supplier, and/or
- In the relevant Australian Standard; and

- Safe working practices and procedures to follow when the equipment is being used.

Ongoing Training

Ongoing or refresher training should be provided periodically to ensure that personal protective equipment is continuing to be used properly. Training should also be provided to workers when work practices and/or equipment are up-dated.

4.4.4 Maintenance and Care of PPE

An effective system of maintenance of PPE is essential to make sure the equipment continues to provide the degree of protection for which it is designed. Therefore, the manufacturer's maintenance schedule (including recommended replacement periods and shelf lives) must always be followed. Inspect PPE before each use. With most PPE, it only takes a few minutes to inspect the equipment for any breaks, tears and visible signs of stress or damage. Maintenance may include: cleaning, examination, replacement, repair and testing. You may be able to carry out simple maintenance (e.g. cleaning), but more intricate repairs must only be carried out by management responsibility to ensure that correct PPE is available and a program is in place. When considering arrangements for providing replacement PPE it must be remembered that unless a task requiring PPE can be stopped, avoided or delayed until new PPE is obtained, replacement PPE must always be readily available.

There should be adequate maintenance of PPE to ensure it controls the risk. Maintenance should include regular visual inspection before each use to determine if the equipment has sustained any damage and that it will work as intended. Where PPE is damaged, so that it may not provide the necessary protection, it should be either repaired or disposed of appropriately and replaced.

The PPE must be inspected for defects every time it is put on. Look for symmetry; does each side look like a mirror image of the other or is one side distorted? Are there any broken, bent, frayed or torn pieces? Are the lenses scratched so they are hard to see through? Is the elastic still springy or is it stretched out? It should also be clean. If it's dirty, clean it with warm soap and water. Don't use solvents or abrasives to clean it. Store it out of sunlight in an area where it will be protected and kept clean.

Replace reusable PPE every 2-5 years, earlier if recommended by the manufacturer or if there is a major impact. Replace any defective parts with parts made by the same manufacturer for that equipment. Do not make makeshift repairs. If it can't be repaired properly, replace it. Don't use paint or glue. Use decals or stickers to mark it.

Helmet is one of the most important items of personal protective equipment used by workers for protection against head injuries which may be caused by falling objects in many industries, for example, mining, tunnelling, quarrying, ship building, construction projects and similar occupations. Head injuries caused by falling objects are usually serious and sometimes fatal. 'This standard has been prepared for industrial safety helmets capable of providing adequate protection from falling objects and other hazards commonly met with in many industries.

4.4.5 Testing Procedures and Standards

Safety Helmet

- Brim - The rimsurrounding the shell
- Chinstrap - An adjustable strap that fits under the chin to secure the helmet Oil the head. Harness -- 'I 'he complete assembly by means of which the helmet is maintained in position on the head, which includes headband, cradle, etc.
- Headband - Part of harness surrounding the head. The plane of lower margin of headband shall correspond to reference line of the head form.
- Anti-Concussion Tapes - Supporting straps which form the cradle.
- Cradle - The fixed or adjustable assembly comparing of anti-concussion tapes and nape strap where provided.
- Nape Strap - An adjustable (with respect to the shell) strap that fits behind the head to secure the helmet and may be integral part of the headband.
- Peak - 'I 'his extension of the shell above the eyes.

- Shell - The hard smoothly finished material that provides the general outer form of the helmet.
- Ventilation Holes - Holes provided in the shell to permit circulation of air-inside the helmet.
- Shock Absorption Resistance - Helmets shall be tested for shock absorption by the method specified. within one minute after subjecting them to the conditions specified in (a), (b) and (c) below: a) A temperature of 50 ± Sock for 4 hours in an oven, h) A temperature of - 10 ± 2° for 4 hours in a refrigerator) and c) "Water flowing over the whole outer surface of the shell at room temperature for 4 hours at a rate of I l/min. No single helmet shall, however, he subjected to more than one of these conditions. The shell shall not show any penetration and/or cracks (separation of material) and harness shall not show any damage deteriorating its function. The force transmitted from the head form to the base shall not be higher than 5 ken(510kef).
- Penetration Resistance - Helmet shall be tested for penetration resistance in accordance with the method specified. Within one minute after subjecting it to one of the conditions given above which has given worst result in shock absorption. These shall neither break nor be pierced through sufficiently to touch the head form; no integral part shall fail or stretch permitting the helmet to be forced down over the head form. The static measurement of the depth of a penetration or dent including the thickness of the material of the shell shall not exceed 10 mm,
- Flammability Resistance - Helmet shell shall be tested for flammability resistance in accordance with the method specified. The material of the shell shall not burn with emission of flame after a period of 5 seconds following removal of flame.
- Electrical Resistance - Helmet shell shall be tested for electrical resistance in accordance with the method specified, and shall not show a leakage current in excess of 3 m A.
- Water Absorption - Helmet shell shall be tested for water absorption in accordance with the method specified, and shall not absorb water more than 5 percent of its mass.

- Heat Resistance - Helmet shell shall be tested for heat resistance in accordance with method specified, and the shell shall not separate, distort or soften.

Method of Testing Sterilization

Procedure: Subject the entire helmet to treatment set out in both (a) anti (b) given below and after treatment examine it for evidence of deterioration, distortion or separation: a) Expose the helmet to a moist atmosphere of antiseptic gas, preferably formaldehyde, at a temperature of25°C for a period of 10 minutes.

METHOD OF TESTING CORROSION RESISTANCE OF METAL PARTS SAMPLES: The samples shall be selected

Procedure

Spray the specimens with a solution of 5 parts of sodium chloride to 95 parts of distilled water (by mass) at room temperature (25°C to 35°C) for a continuous period of 24 hours. Then wash the parts in clean running water, and dry. Inspect for signs of corrosion.

METHOD OF CHECKING CLEARANCE ABOVE THE HEAD AND THE WEARING HEIGHT (DEPTH OF FIT)

Clearance above the Head

In the case of helmet which has reinforcing ribs, measure the depth of rib and correct the measured clearance accordingly. Mount the helmet on a head form (see IS: 7692-1975*) corresponding to the size of headband marked on the helmet, in a position similar to that which it would occupy on a man's head. Apply a load of 10 kg, to the top of the helmet (this can be conveniently applied by using a 10 kg bag of sand). Measure the clearance by means of a rod of diameter not more than 10 mm inserted through the whole dri1Jed in the vertical axis of the head form.

Wearing Height (Depth Of Fit)

Mount the helmet on a head form corresponding to the size of headband marked on the helmet and apply a pressure of 10 kg. Mark on the head form the position of the lower edge of the headband. Remove the helmet and measure the vertical distance between the top of the head form and the mark showing the position occupied by the headband.

Shock Absorption Test

Samples: The samples shall be selected. A wooden head form (set IS: 7692- 1975*) shall be used. A Gauge and Recording Apparatus for Measuring Force - The gauge and the associated recording apparatus shall have proper time constant to be able to measure the impact loading up to 40 ken (4080 kef) independent of the time of application of the force and a slow application of the load required for its calibration. The gauge shall have a minimum stiffness of 500 kingthe head form shall be mounted on the gauge so that its vertical axis through the crown coincides with the vertical axis of the gauge.

- Accuracy - The overall accuracy of the recording apparatus shall be 10 percent.
- Block - Concrete or similar monolithic block to support the gauge and head form, having the minimum dimensions: height I'm, length 1 m, width 0'6 m and mass 1 t. The block shall be bedded on dry sand on a solid floor.
- Striker - A striker in the form of a rectangular block of wood weighing 3 kg and having a horizontal striking face 180 mm X 180 rom. The striker shall slide freely and without oscillation down two vertical guide wires so positioned that the centre of gravity of the striker lies on the vertical axis of the gauge and both lie in the plane of the guide wires.

Method of Testing Penetration Resistance

Procedure

Mount helmet on any head form (see IS: 7692-1975*). Drop freely a plumb bob of 500 g mass with a conical steel point having an included angle of 360 and a spherical point radius of not more than 0·5 mm from a clear height of 3'0 m with the pointed end downwards on to the top of the crown of the helmet. Examine the helmet for piercing or denting, failure of any integral parts, etc.

Method of Testing Flammability Resistance

The fol1owing accessories shall be used with the burner: a) Reservoir, b) Connecting tube of polyethylene or soft rubber, c) Absolute alcohol (ethanol), d) Copper wire 0'71 mm diameter having a free length of not less than 100 mm, and e) Stand to help the reservoir.

The absolute alcohol shall be filled in the reservoir and the tube air bubbles entrapped in the tube shall be removed by pressing the tube several times. Cotton waste soaked in spirit shall be kept in the cup on the burner an n d lighted. After a few minutes when the burner is sufficiently heated the regulator of burner shall be turned to allow the spirit to flow in the form of vapour.

Burner shall be operated with the valve so as to get a flame height of 150 Hun. Level of the fuel shall be not Jess than 760 mm above the base of the burner. Satisfactory operation of burner shall be checked by inserting in the flame the bare copper wires in position normally occupied by low edge of the test piece, that is, 50 mm above the burner and reaching farther edge of the flame. The wire should not take I110rC than 6 seconds to melt.

- Safety suit: Materials of Construction Many different materials of construction are available for various protective body garments.
- Paper-like fiber used for disposable suits provide protection against dust and small splashes.
- Treated wool and cotton adapts well to changing temperatures, is comfortable, fire-resistant and protects against dust, abrasions, and rough and irritating surfaces.
- Duck is a closely woven cotton fabric that protects against cuts and bruises when handling heavy, sharp, or rough materials.
- Leather is often used to protect against dry heat and flames.
- Rubber, rubberized fabrics, neoprene and plastics protect against certain chemical and physical hazards. When chemical or physical hazards are present, check with the

clothing manufacturer to ensure that the material selected will provide protection against the specific hazard. Typical Laboratory Operations In a typical laboratory setting where small containers of biological agents, radioactive materials, or hazardous chemicals are handled, a lab coat is the minimum required body protection. In this type of setting, potential for contact with significant quantities of hazardous materials/agents is relatively low. Lab coats protect the body against incidental exposure to hazardous agents and minimize potential for "transferring" hazardous agents to other areas through contaminated clothing.

- Lab coats should be flame retardant if there is risk of fire due to open flames or chemical reaction.
- When working with pathogenic organisms, a rear-closing gown may be more appropriate rather than a lab coat. Greater detail regarding PPE for biological agent protection is provided in the EHS Bio safety in the BSL-2 Laboratory and Blood borne Pathogens (including HIV/HBV/HCV) web-based training modules and associated Safe Operating Procedures, available through the EHS web site. Protection from Chemicals In situations where the potential for chemical contact is greater than incidental, specialized chemical-resistant clothing is appropriate. Selection of the proper chemical resistant clothing must consider:
- Body part(s) that could be exposed. This information will assist in the selection of the proper style. Full body coverage is necessary if there is potential for large splashes that could impact the legs, arms, and torso. If exposure potential is limited, then an apron, sleeves, or jacket may be sufficient.
- Physical state of the chemical contaminant. The highest level of skin protection is afforded with a fully-encapsulated suit. This type of suit is impermeable to gases and vapors' and protects all parts of the body (hands, arms, head, face, torso, legs, etc.). A fully-encapsulated suit looks like a space suit. NOTE: No UNL employee is authorized to conduct tasks or enter atmospheres where a fully-encapsulated suit is necessary.

- Non-encapsulating suits, jackets, aprons, and coveralls (depending on the body parts exposed) are appropriate to protect against liquid splashes and dusts/particulates. Non-encapsulating protection does not fully cover the wearer and has separate gloves and footwear even if a full body suit is used.
- Permeability and penetration with respect to the classes of chemicals of concern. The material of construction is an important consideration when selecting an encapsulating garment since different types of fabric/coatings have differing resistance to various chemicals (permeability). In addition, seams, openings, and fabric imperfections also influence the protectiveness of a garment (penetration data).
- Similar to the approach taken with gloves, manufacturers will often test their products. Using the results of these tests, the manufacturer will provide recommendations for their products based on the types of chemical and physical state of the contaminants of concern.

High Visibility

Body protection garments are available to enhance a person's visibility (e.g., workers in construction zones, traffic controllers, etc.). There are two common ANSI standards associated with high visibility (HV) clothing, ANSI 107 and ANSI 207. When high visibility clothing is needed, choose clothing that meets the applicable ANSI standard or other national or international consensus standard.

Welding

Welding aprons, sleeves, bibs, and coats are available to protect against hot splashes from molten metals. The authority mandating welding protective clothing is ANSI Z49.1, Safety in Welding, Cutting, and Allied Processes. However, this standard does not incorporate specific garment test protocols like it does for welding helmets and protective eyewear. Rather, it states: "Clothing shall provide sufficient coverage, and be made of suitable materials, to minimize skin burns caused by sparks, spatter, or radiation." Heavier materials such as woollen clothing or heavy cotton are preferable to lighter materials because they are more difficult to ignite. Cotton clothing, if used for protection, should be chemically treated to reduce its combustibility. Flame resistance should conform to the minimum specifications of ASTM D6413, NFPA 2112, or equivalent.

Chainsaws

In the United States, the primary performance standard for chainsaw protective clothing is ASTM F1897, Standard Specification for Leg Protection for Chain Saw Users. When selecting leg protection for chainsaw use, select a manufacturer that adheres to this standard or an equivalent international consensus standard.

Cut-resistance

Clothing to help protect against cuts can be made from a variety of materials. Most often, this type of clothing is not associated with any particular performance standard. Thus, selection is largely based on good judgment. In some cases, such as typical kitchen operations, sufficient protection may be afforded by a heavy apron. However, in a meat-packing-like operation Kevlar or stainless steel mesh may be more appropriate. The key is to select a product that is well matched to the risk.

CHAPTER 5

Housekeeping

5.1 Introduction to Housekeeping and Maintenance

By definition housekeeping means having place for everything and everything in its place in proper order. Housekeeping standard reflects an Organization's work culture. Poor housekeeping contributes to accidents, fires and poor work environment. Good housekeeping is only achieved by proper planning. This includes

- A Well Planned Layout
- Orderly Arrangement of Equipment
- Systematic Material Storage
- Stacking and Movement
- Efficient Waste Disposal
- Day to Day Maintenance of Cleanliness and Tidiness

Good layout would means proper position of buildings, plant, machinery and other materials permitting the most efficient utilization of materials, processes and methods.

5S

5S is a systematic approach to work place organization, But it's also much more than that. 5S is about efficiency, competitiveness and survival. It is a deceptively simple system that creates an organized and productive workplace.

But it's not just about cleaning up and eliminating toolboxes. 5S creates a workplace environment that can adapt and succeed in this turbulent times. Chaos and unproductively are your enemies; Organization and efficiency are your allies

If implemented correctly and followed diligently, 5S will lead to:

- Lower costs
- Better quality
- Improved safety
- Increased productivity
- Higher employee satisfaction

5S is sometimes called the five pillars because just like the physical pillars that hold up a structure, 5S has five elements that support the effectiveness of the system. And just like the pillars of a building, if one was to weaken or fail, the entire structure could be greatly compromised

5S is a system, a philosophy and a culture. The true power of 5S reveals itself when the whole organization embraces its ideals and its employees see that the business is transforming itself.

The 5S model for workplace efficiency and organization is both powerful and simple. It has the potential to transform the company into a safe and productive warehouse, manufacturing facility or office.

5.2 Importance of Good Housekeeping

Effective housekeeping can eliminate some workplace hazards and help get a job done safely and properly. Poor housekeeping can frequently contribute to accidents by hiding hazards that cause injuries. If the sight of paper, debris, clutter and spills is accepted as normal, then other more serious health and safety hazards may be taken for granted.

Housekeeping is not just cleanliness. It includes keeping work areas neat and orderly; maintaining halls and floors free of slip and trip hazards; and removing of waste materials (e.g., paper, cardboard) and other fire hazards from work areas. It also requires paying attention to important details such as the layout of the whole workplace, aisle marking, the adequacy of storage facilities, and maintenance. Good housekeeping is also a basic part of accident and fire prevention.

Effective housekeeping is an ongoing operation: it is not a hit-and-miss clean-up done occasionally. Periodic "panic" clean-ups are costly and ineffective in reducing accidents.

5.2.1 Purpose of Workplace Housekeeping

Poor housekeeping can be a cause of accidents, such as:

- tripping over loose objects on floors, stairs and platforms
- being hit by falling objects
- slipping on greasy, wet or dirty surfaces
- striking against projecting, poorly stacked items or misplaced material
- cutting, puncturing, or tearing the skin of hands or other parts of the body on projecting nails, wire or steel strapping

To avoid these hazards, a workplace must "maintain" order throughout a workday. Although this effort requires a great deal of management and planning, the benefits are many.

5.2.2 Planning of Good Housekeeping Programme

A good housekeeping program plans and manages the orderly storage and movement of materials from point of entry to exit. It includes a material flow plan to ensure minimal handling. The plan also ensures that work areas are not used as storage areas by having workers move materials to and from work areas as needed. Part of the plan could include investing in extra bins and more frequent disposal.

The costs of this investment could be offset by the elimination of repeated handling of the same material and more effective use of the workers' time. Often, ineffective or insufficient storage planning results in materials being handled and stored in hazardous ways. Knowing the plant layout and the movement of materials throughout the workplace can help plan work procedures.

Worker training is an essential part of any good housekeeping program.

Workers need to know how to work safely with the products they use. They also need to know how to protect other workers such as by posting signs (e.g., "Wet - Slippery Floor") and reporting any unusual conditions.

Housekeeping order is "maintained" not "achieved." Cleaning and organization must be done regularly, not just at the end of the shift. Integrating housekeeping into jobs can help ensure this is done. A good housekeeping program identifies and assigns responsibilities for the following:

- clean up during the shift
- day-to-day clean-up
- waste disposal
- removal of unused materials
- inspection to ensure clean-up is complete

Do not forget out-of-the-way places such as shelves, basements, sheds, and boiler rooms that would otherwise be overlooked. The orderly arrangement of operations, tools, equipment and supplies is an important part of a good housekeeping program.

The final addition to any housekeeping program is inspection. It is the only way to check for deficiencies in the program so that changes can be made. The documents on workplace inspection checklists provide a general guide and examples of checklists for inspecting offices and manufacturing facilities.

5.2.3 Elements of an Effective Housekeeping Program

Dust and Dirt Removal

In some jobs, enclosures and exhaust ventilation systems may fail to collect dust, dirt and chips adequately. Vacuum cleaners are suitable for removing light dust and dirt. Industrial models have special fittings for cleaning walls, ceilings, ledges, machinery, and other hard-to-reach places where dust and dirt may accumulate.

Special-purpose vacuums are useful for removing hazardous substances. For example, vacuum cleaners fitted with HEPA (high efficiency particulate air) filters may be used to capture fine particles of asbestos or fibre glass.

Dampening (wetting) floors or using sweeping compounds before sweeping reduces the amount of airborne dust. The dust and grime that collect in places like shelves, piping, conduits, light fixtures, reflectors, windows, cupboards and lockers may require manual cleaning. Compressed air should not be used for removing dust, dirt or chips from equipment or work surfaces.

Employee Facilities

Employee facilities need to be adequate, clean and well maintained. Lockers are necessary for storing employees' personal belongings. Washroom facilities require cleaning once or more each shift. They also need to have a good supply of soap, towels plus disinfectants, if needed.

If workers are using hazardous materials, employee facilities should provide special precautions such as showers, washing facilities and change rooms. Some facilities may require two locker rooms with showers between. Using such double locker rooms allows workers to shower off workplace contaminants and prevents them from contaminating their "street clothes" by keeping their work clothes separated from the clothing that they wear home.

Smoking, eating or drinking in the work area should be prohibited where toxic materials are handled. The eating area should be separate from the work area and should be cleaned properly each shift.

Surfaces

Floors: Poor floor conditions are a leading cause of accidents so cleaning up spilled oil and other liquids at once is important. Allowing chips, shavings and dust to accumulate can also cause accidents. Trapping chips, shavings and dust before they reach the floor or cleaning them up regularly can prevent their accumulation. Areas that cannot be cleaned continuously, such as entrance ways, should have anti-slip flooring. Keeping floors in good order also means replacing any worn, ripped, or damaged flooring that poses a tripping hazard.

Walls

Light-coloured walls reflect light while dirty or dark-coloured walls absorb light. Contrasting colours warn of physical hazards and mark obstructions such as pillars. Paint can highlight railings, guards and other safety equipment, but should never be used as a substitute for guarding. The program should outline the regulations and standards for colours.

Maintain Light Fixtures

Dirty light fixtures reduce essential light levels. Clean light fixtures can improve lighting efficiency significantly.

Aisles and Stairways

Aisles should be wide enough to accommodate people and vehicles comfortably and safely. Aisle space allows for the movement of people, products and materials. Warning signs and mirrors can improve sight-lines in blind corners. Arranging aisles properly encourages people to use them so that they do not take shortcuts through hazardous areas.

Keeping aisles and stairways clear is important. They should not be used for temporary "overflow" or "bottleneck" storage. Stairways and aisles also require adequate lighting.

Spill Control

The best way to control spills is to stop them before they happen. Regularly cleaning and maintaining machines and equipment is one way. Another is to use drip pans and guards where possible spills might occur. When spills do occur, it is important to clean them up immediately. Absorbent materials are useful for wiping up greasy, oily or other liquid spills. Used absorbents must be disposed of properly and safely.

Tools and Equipment

Tool housekeeping is very important, whether in the tool room, on the rack, in the yard, or on the bench. Tools require suitable fixtures with marked locations to provide orderly arrangement, both in the tool room and near the work bench. Returning them promptly after use reduces the chance of being misplaced or lost. Workers should regularly inspect, clean and repair all tools and take any damaged or worn tools out of service

Maintenance

The maintenance of buildings and equipment may be the most important element of good housekeeping. Maintenance involves keeping buildings, equipment and machinery in safe, efficient working order and in good repair. This includes maintaining sanitary facilities and regularly painting and cleaning walls. Broken windows, damaged doors, defective plumbing and broken floor surfaces can make a workplace look neglected; these conditions can cause accidents and affect work practices. So it is important to replace or fix broken or damaged items as quickly as possible. A good maintenance program provides for the inspection, maintenance, upkeep and repair of tools, equipment, machines and processes.

Waste Disposal

The regular collection, grading and sorting of scrap contribute to good housekeeping practices. It also makes it possible to separate materials that can be recycled from those going to waste disposal facilities.

Allowing material to build up on the floor wastes time and energy since additional time is required for cleaning it up. Placing scrap containers near where the waste is produced encourages orderly waste disposal and makes collection easier. All waste receptacles should be clearly labelled (e.g., recyclable glass, plastic, scrap metal, etc.).

Storage

Good organization of stored materials is essential for overcoming material storage problems whether on a temporary or permanent basis. There will also be fewer strain injuries if the amount of handling is reduced, especially if less manual materials handling is required. The location of the stockpiles should not interfere with work but they should still be readily available when required. Stored materials should allow at least one metre (or about three feet) of clear space under sprinkler heads.

Stacking cartons and drums on a firm foundation and cross tying them, where necessary, reduces the chance of their movement. Stored materials should not obstruct aisles, stairs, exits, fire equipment, emergency eyewash fountains, emergency showers, or first aid stations. All storage areas should be clearly marked.

Flammable, combustible, toxic and other hazardous materials should be stored in approved containers in designated areas that are appropriate for the different hazards that they pose. Storage of materials should meet all requirements specified in the fire codes and the regulations of environmental and occupational health and safety agencies in your jurisdiction.

5.3 Understanding Housekeeping Responsibilities

- Organize, supervise and coordinate the work of housekeeping staff on day- to day basis.
- Ensure excellence in housekeeping sanitation, safety, comfort and aesthetics for hotel guests.

- Prepare duty rosters and supervise the discipline and conduct of her staff.
- Ensure proper communication within the department by conducting regular meeting with the staff.
- Recruit new employees and train them for the housekeeping jobs.
- Counsel and motivate employees on various duties.
- Establish and maintain standard operating procedures for cleaning and develop new procedures to increase efficiency of labour and product use.
- Search and test new techniques and products in the market.
- Maintain regular inventory and checking of furniture, linen, uniform, equipment's in the hotel.
- Evaluate employee performance for promotions and transfers.
- Approval of supply requisitions for the housekeeping and to maintain minimum stock and cost control procedures for all materials.
- Check the reports, files, registers maintained in the department.
- Provide budget to the management and control of budgets

5.4 Develop Good Housekeeping Habits

- Sweep smaller debris such as broken glass, nails and other trash into a dustpan, before placing it into the trashcan.
- If sharp objects such as nails, broken glass or metal fall onto the floor, use leather gloves in addition to using the dustpan and broom to dispose of the trash.
- Trashcans should be emptied into dumpsters frequently so that they do not become too heavy
- Keeping tools and equipment clean and properly stored when not in use.
- Wrapping up and storing hoses, cables and wires when not in use
- Developing good housekeeping habits will protect you and your co-workers from injuries on the job.

- Make time for housekeeping tasks on a daily basis. Set aside a little time during the workday and at the end of your shift for housekeeping.
    - Evaluate your workspace before starting work. Look for slip, trip, and fall hazards, fire hazards, machine hazards, cut hazards, and so forth.
- Remove those hazards before starting work. Clean up spills. Put away tools and electrical cords you don't need. Close drawers. Clean up waste materials and dispose of them properly.
- Don't leave equipment running when you leave the work area. Turn it off and clean it up so that it is ready for the next time it's used.
- Clean up as you go. Put tools and equipment away in their proper place when you are through with them. Waiting until the end of the shift exposes you and others to trip hazards all day.
    - And finally, take responsibility for hazards even if you didn't create the hazard or it's not in your work area. Eliminate or report all hazards
- Be sure to clean up spills of water, oil, or other liquids. Paper towels can be used for water. Oil and other chemicals may require special absorbent wipes. For some hazardous chemicals, special training and equipment are required to clean up spills.
- Liquid leaks must be repaired right away. If you can't do it safely yourself, report the problem immediately and place a barrier around the affected area to prevent slips.
- Pick objects off the floor. Plastic on a concrete floor, for instance, can be very hazardous. Even a small piece, which can be hard to see, can send somebody tumbling to the floor.
    - Sweep up debris and waste materials. Some granular particles can act just like liquid spills on the floor and cause a slip and fall.
- And don't forget to wear slip-resistant shoes to help prevent a fall should you encounter a slippery surface.
- Clean up debris such as straps and bands from boxes that can become entangled in a person's legs.

- Put away electrical cords and air hoses when not in use. And even when using them, be careful where you place them. Make sure it's not somewhere somebody could trip over them.
- Don't stack boxes or other items in walkways.
- Keep drawers closed so that someone doesn't come by and tumble over an open drawer.
  - Be careful when you carry objects. Make sure you can see where you're going and watch out for obstacles that could cause a trip.
- Put away tools and other production equipment after use. Leaving items lying around on the floor could cause someone to trip and fall.
- Evaluate your workspace
- Remove hazards before starting work
- Turn equipment off after using it
- Clean up as you go
- Never ignore a safety hazard
- Good housekeeping helps prevent workplace fires and accidents
- Keep alert to housekeeping hazards
- Eliminate or report hazards you identify anywhere in the facility
- Eliminates accident and fire hazards
- Maintains safe, healthy work conditions
- Saves time, money, materials, space, and effort
- Improves productivity and quality
- Boosts morale
- Reflects a well-run organization

GOOD
HOUSEKEEPING
IS THE
KEY TO SAFETY
• CLEANLINESS
• ORDER
• A PLACE FOR
EVERYTHING
ARE ESSENTIALS
OF SAFETY

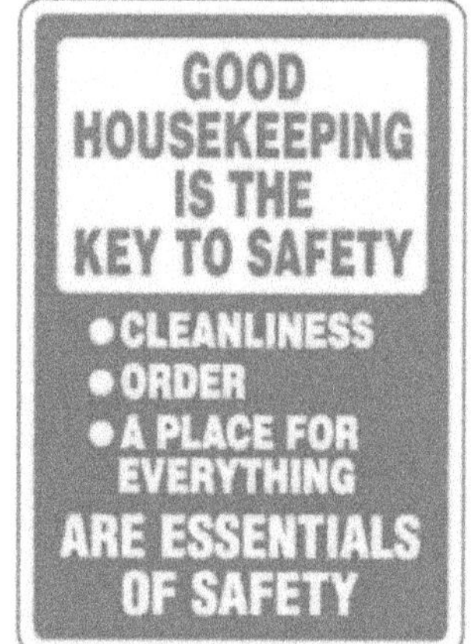

5.5 Benefits of Good Housekeeping

Good housekeeping at work places benefits not only the but also the employee. Good housekeeping practices generally reflect good management practices and pride in the workplace, signalling that the company cares about safety. The benefits of following good housekeeping are as follows

Order: Eliminate clutter which is a common cause of accidents, such as slips, trips, and falls, and fire and explosions.

Protection: Reduce the chances of harmful materials entering the body (e.g., dusts, vapours).

Productivity: Improve productivity as the right tools and materials for the job will be easy to find.

Impression: Improve your company's image as good housekeeping reflects a well-run business. An orderly workplace will impress all who enter it – employees, visitors, customers, etc.

Inventory: Help your company to keep its inventory to a minimum as good housekeeping makes it easier to keep an accurate count of inventories.

Space: Help your company to make the best use of its space

Work place: Make the workplace neat, comfortable and pleasant – not a dangerous eyesore

Ease of flow: Reduced handling to ease the flow of materials

Fire: Decreased fire hazards

Efficiency: More efficient equipment clean-up and maintenance

Hygiene: Better hygienic conditions leading to improved health

Property Damage: Reduced property damage by improving preventive maintenance

Hazardous Substance: Reduces exposure to hazardous substances;

Others: Sufficient waste management programme, less janitorial work an improved moral.

Benefits of Good Housekeeping

Area	Benefit
Productivity	Waste reduction through systematic work systems
Quality	Fewer human errors through visual control and other systems
Equipment performance	Routine cleaning and inspection prevent unscheduled breakdowns
Safety	Reduction of hazards through proper storage and organization of items in the workplace

5.6 Cost of Poor Housekeeping

Poor housekeeping contributes to accidents by hiding hazards that cause injuries. Worksites that have poor housekeeping practices with rubbish, waste and broken items around the grounds and a general appearance of poor maintenance do not instill confidence in consumers about the products produced on site. Poor housekeeping practices may cause accidents in the workplace and/or provide fuel for fires.

Poor housekeeping practices may lead to slips, trips and falls. These accidents may be the result of

- poor maintenance practices
- inadequate cleaning practices
- cracked and uneven floors
- Work areas and walkways blocked by waste, equipment, unused items, broken items etc.
- spills
- hoses and equipment lying around
- product overflow
- waste that hasn't been disposed of
- items that haven't been put away
- inadequate storage facilities
- rubbish that hasn't been disposed off
- broken items such broken pallets stacked up against the walls

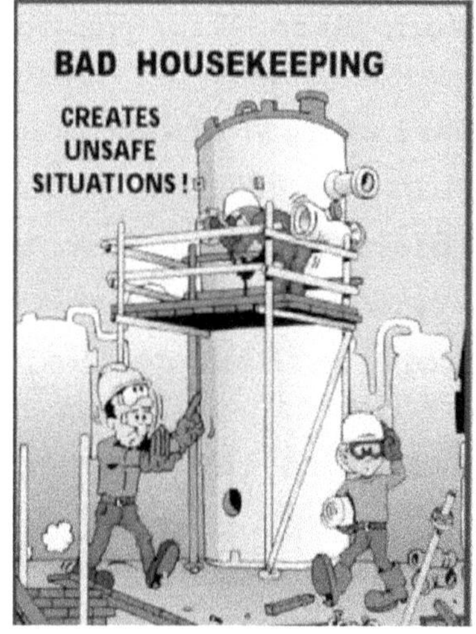

- Tools not properly stored are more easily damaged
- Time is wasted cleaning up or looking for items lost in the mess
- Garbage area attract rodents and insects and can create health hazards with high level of bacteria
- Emergency exits and access to fire extinguishers can be blocked

- Sharp objects, wires, greases, scrap materials and lumber without protruding nails are among the typical workplace hazards
- Fire safety is reduced with proper storage of materials

Role of Supervisor in reducing Poor Housekeeping

- Ensuring the work area you are responsible for is maintained in a tidy condition
- Ensuring workplace policies and procedures for housekeeping practices are in place and being followed
- Ensuring all your workers are appropriately trained and follow good housekeeping policy and procedures
- Ensuring any incidents relating to poor housekeeping are reported, you investigate the incident quickly and take any actions to prevent the incident happening again
- Conducting regular inspections of your work area including cleanliness of floors, correct storage of equipment, hoses, waste bins are routinely emptied to prevent buildup etc.

5.7 Basics of 5S

5S is amongst the first and fundamental steps implemented by an enterprise towards the path of implementing Total Quality Management & continuous improvement at the operational level. 5S is a process designed to organize the workplace, keep it clean, and maintain effective & standard conditions. It installs the discipline required to enable each individual to achieve & maintain a world class environment.

The use of this tool was started in 1972 by Henry Ford in United States as the CANDO programme Cleaning up, Arranging, Neatness, Discipline & Ongoing improvement. The technique was popularized as Japanese 5S in 1980 by Hiroyuki Hirano.

Many Enterprises have practiced the 5S & derived significant benefits from it. In particular, the technique has been widely practiced in Japan. Most Japanese 5S practitioners considered 5S useful not just for improving their thinking processes too. In Japan it is called " Workplace Management". 5S will be needed if the workplace is messy & unorganized. It will also be needed if employees spend extra time in searching tools, papers, Information's, etc.

Meaning of 5S

5S is the acronym for five Japanese words; Seiri, Seiton, Sieso, Seiketsu, Shitsuke & they represent the five steps for systematic technique for good housekeeping as indicated in the table below:

Table 5.1 The five steps of Japanese 5S

Seiri (Sort)	Distinguish between necessary &Unnecessary items. Remove the latter.
Seiton (Set in order)	Enforce the dictum 'a place for everything & everything in its place'.
Seiso (Shine)	Clean up the workplace & look for ways to keep it clean.
Seiketsu (Standardize)	Maintain & monitor adherence to the first three S's.
Shitsuke (Sustain)	Follow the rule to keep the workplace 5S-Right. Hold the gain.

Why do we practice 5s?

The General concept of the 5S is that they are intended to eliminate waste.

Working in disorder is neither productive, nor safe. 5S is a simple & practical method to install a quality culture at the work place. It is relatively easy to undertake, & requires minimal addition resources. The first and small investment made in time & effort pays off in a much bigger manner when the results are realized & maintained.

- Among the benefits of implementing 5S are:
- workplace becomes cleaner, safer, well organized & more pleasant
- Floor space utilization is improved
- Workflow becomes smoother & more systematic & non value added activities are reduced;
- Time for searching tools, materials and document is minimized
- Machine breakdowns are reduced since clean and well-maintained equipment breaks down less frequently and it also becomes easier to diagnose and repair before breakdowns occur, therefore extending equipment life;
- Errors are minimized leading to making defect-free products;
- consumables and material wastage are minimized;
- The morale and satisfaction of employees improves; and

- The productivity of the organization improves together with the quality of products and services.

The 5 S
SORT / CLEARING
Throw away unnecessary and unrelated materials in your workplace.
SET / ORGANIZE
Set everything in proper place for quick retrieval and storage
SHINE & SWEEP
Clean the workplace; everyone should be a janitor
STANDARDIZE
Standardize the way of maintaining order and cleanliness
SUSTAIN
Practice '5 S' daily - make it a way of life; this also means 'commitment'

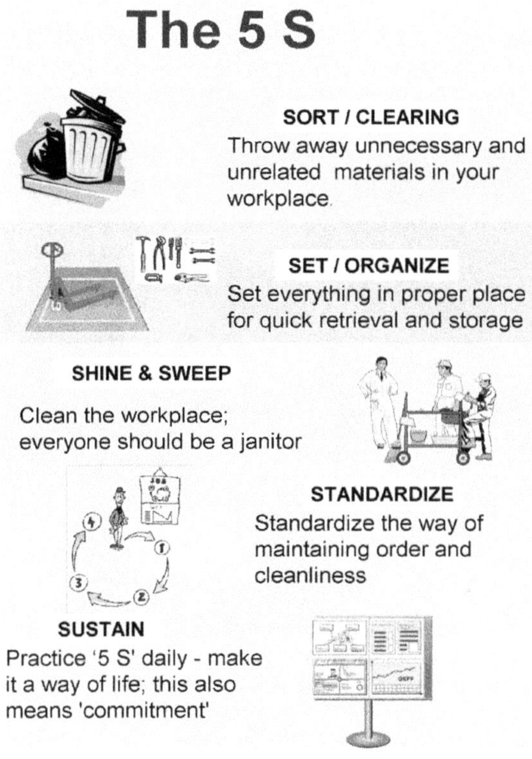

Fig. 5.1 Disorder is neither productive nor safe

Practicing the 5S Technique

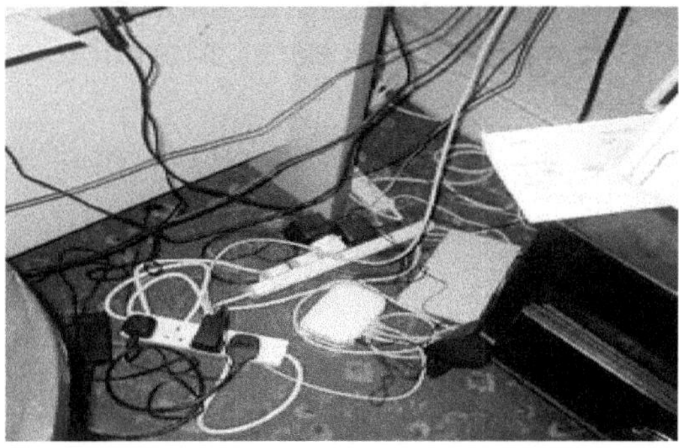

The meaning, methods of implementing and benefits of each of the 5S are given below.

Sort – Seiri

The emphasis of Seiri is on stratification management and being able to spot the unwanted and unnecessary before they become problematic.

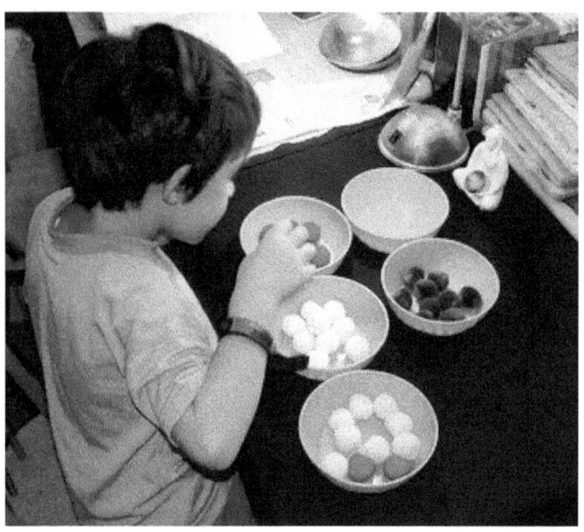

Fig. 5.2 Sort – Seiri

It means distinguishing or sort out between 'wanted' and 'unwanted items' at place of work and removal of unwanted item.

Methods

- First decide what is necessary and what is unnecessary. To find out unnecessary items you should not only check the floor but also shelves, lockers, storehouse, stairs, roofs, notice boards, etc.
- Put a red tag on unnecessary items and keep them in a separate area.
- Discard or throw those items which have not been used in the past one year.
- Things used once in 6 to 12 months may be stored at a distance from work station.
- Things used more than once a month should be available at a central point in the workplace.

- Things used hourly/everyday/once a week should be near the work station or may be worn by or kept in the pocket of your worker there.

Benefits

- Your useful floor is saved.
- Your searching time of tools, materials, and papers is reduced.
- You have better flow of work.
- Your inventory cost of unnecessary items is reduced.

Set in Order – Seiton

Seiton in essence can be defined as neatness, having things in the right places or set up so that they are readily available for use, eliminating the need to search. Once everything has a right place so that it's functionally placed for quality and safety, it can then be deemed that the workplace is neat. While Seiri helps you to decide what items are needed, Seiton helps you to decide the way things are to be placed.

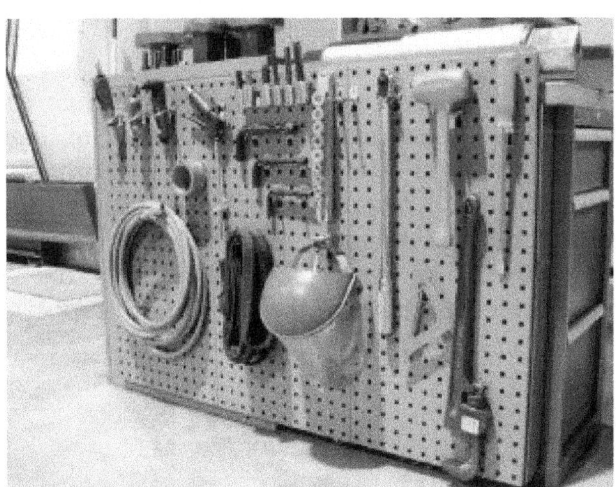

Fig. 5.3 Seiton

- It is arranging items in such a manner that they are easy to use.
- Labelling them so that they are easy to find and put back.
- This means a place for everything (necessary) and everything in its place. No more homeless items.

Methods

- If necessary, reassign spaces, racks, cabinets, etc.
- Decide the right places for everything.
- Put all materials and equipment at a place allocated to them with proper label or signalization. Use alerts or indications for out-of stock situations.
- Use floor paint marking to define working area, path, entrance/exit, safety equipment, cart/ trolley locations, etc.
- Use standard colour coding for pipelines for steam, water, gas, drainage, etc.
- Use display cautions, messages, instructions at proper place at proper height and written clearly

Benefits

- You take things out and keep things back easily.
- You make lesser mistakes.
- You reduce searching time.
- Your work environment becomes safe

Shine – Seiso

Seiso places emphasis on cleaning so that things are clean; in other words carrying out cleaning as a form of inspection i.e. getting rid of waste, and foreign matter. It is important to note that depending on the circumstance, with higher quality, higher precision and finer processing technologies, even the minute details may have the greatest ramifications, hence the importance to carry out cleaning as a form of inspection.

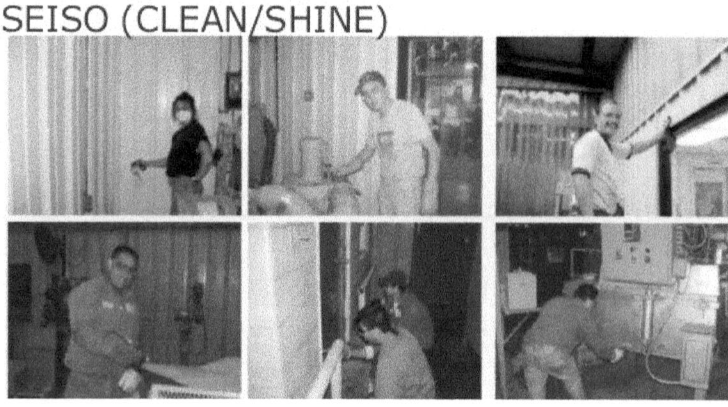

This means removing dirt, strain, filth, soot and dust from the work area.

Methods

- Divide the total area in zones and allocate responsibility for cleaning for each zone.
- Decide on cleaning points, order of cleaning, type of cleaning, cleaning aid required, etc.
- Display cleaning schedule.
- During cleaning look for defective conditions (loose bolts, vibrations, excessive sound, high temperature, fallen tools, etc.) and solve the problem.
- Allocate space for storage of cleaning aids and consumables for cleaning.

Benefits

- Your work place becomes free of dirt and stains which is the starting point for quality.
- Your equipment lifespan will be prolonged and breakdowns will be less.
- Creates a pleasant environment.
- Prevents accidents.

Standardize - Seiketsu

This aspect of the 5S focuses on standardization, making the first three S's, Seiri, Seiton, and Seiso a constant routine. The emphasis here is on visual management, an important aspect to attain and maintain standardized conditions to enable the individuals always act quickly.

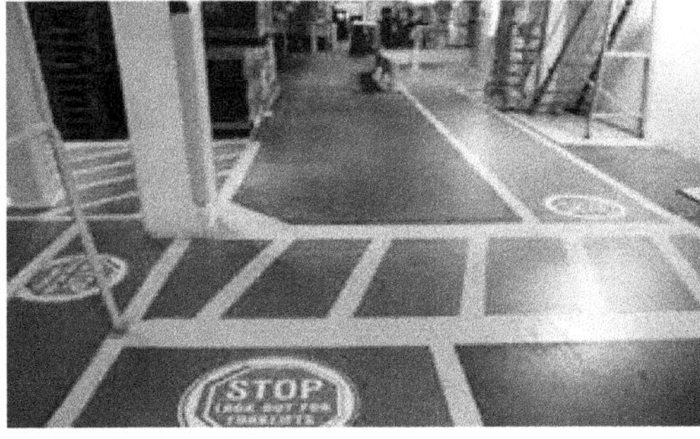

Fig. 5.4 Seiketsu

This call for systematizing the above 4S practices. This means ensuring that whatever cleanliness and orderliness is achieved should be maintained.

Methods

Document procedures and guidelines for sorting, set in order and shine.

- Make a checklist for each section and train your people in using them
- Carry out periodic evaluation by using the above check list.
- Use visual management to act quickly, for example putting/using:
    - Open and shut directional labels on switches, etc.
    - Temperature and safety labels
    - Zone labels on measuring meters (normal zone, danger zone, etc.)
    - OK or hold marks on product.
    - Put transparency control
    - Make transparent covers of drawers.
    - Put inspection windows in the metal covers
    - Use location maps with emergency exits, fire fighting equipment, etc.

Benefits

- Your activities will be simplified.
- You will have consistency in the work practices.
- You will avoid mistakes.
- With better visual and transparency management work efficiency will improve.

Sustain - Shitsuke

Shitsuke places emphasis on being able to forge a workplace with good habits and discipline. Demonstrating to others what needs to be done and encouraging practice amongst them. This is mainly a management responsibility.

Sustain also means 'Discipline'. It denotes your commitment to maintain orderliness and to practice first 3S as a way of life.

This also requires that your employees show positive interest and overcome resistance to change.

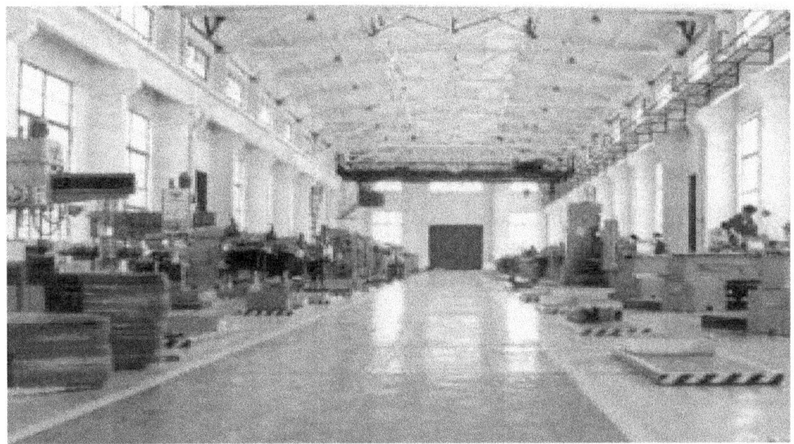

Fig. 5.5 Shitsuke

Methods

- Create awareness and publicize the system. For example develop 5S News, 5S Posters, 5S Slogans, 5S Day, etc.
- Create a structure of how and when 5S activities will be implemented.
- Formulate guidelines for audit/evaluation of 5S implementation.
- Provide management support by providing resources and leadership.
- Reward and recognize best performers.

Benefits

- Promotes habit for complying with workplace rules and procedures.
- Creates healthy atmosphere and a good work place.
- Helps you to develop team work.
- Provides you with data for improving 5S.

Management's role in implementing 5S

It is important to note that the implementation of 5S concerns and benefits everyone in the organization. Like any other initiative, management has the important role to facilitate and support the process by:

- Acknowledging the importance of 5S for the organization;
- Allowing employees time for 5S;
- Providing resources and infrastructure for 5S implementation;
- Personal involvement in implementation of 5S;
- Creating tangible and intangible rewards and recognition for improvements;
- Promoting ongoing 5S effort.

CHAPTER 6

Occupational Health

6.1 Definition

Occupational Health is the promotion and maintenance of the highest degree of physical, mental and social well-being of workers in all OCCUPATIONS by preventing departures from health, controlling risks and the adaption of work to people, and people to their jobs.

6.2 Common Occupational Disease

An "occupational disease" is any disease contracted primarily as a result of an exposure to risk factors arising from work activity. "Work-related diseases" have multiple causes, where factors in the work environment may play a role, together with other risk factors, in the development of such diseases.

In Factories Act, 1948 Schedule III [Sections 89 & 90] modifiable diseases are,

List of modifiable Occupational Diseases

1. Lead poisoning including poisoning by any preparation or compound of lead or their squeal.
2. Lead-tetra-ethyl poisoning.
3. Phosphorus poisoning or its sequelae.
4. Mercury poisoning or its sequelae.
5. Manganese poisoning or its sequelae.
6. Arsenic poisoning or its sequelae.
7. Poisoning by nitrous fumes.
8. Carbon bisulphate poisoning.
9. Benzene poisoning, including poisoning by any of its homologues, their nitro or amide derivatives or its sequelae.

10. Chrome ulceration or its sequelae.
11. Anthrax.
12. Silicosis.
13. Poisoning by halogens or halogen derivatives of the hydrocarbons of the aliphatic series.
14. Pathological manifestations due to-
    (a) Radium or other radioactive substances;
    (b) X-rays.
15. Primary epitheliomatous cancer of the skin.
16. Toxic anaemia.
17. Toxic jaundice due to poisonous substances.
18. Oil acne or dermatitis due to mineral oils and compounds containing mineral oil base.
19. Byssionosis.
20. Asbestosis.
21. Occupational or contact dermatitis caused by direct contact with chemicals and paints. These are of two types, that is, primary irritants and allergic sensitizers.
22. Noise induced hearing loss (exposures to high noise levels).
23. Beryllium poisoning.
24. Carbon monoxide.
25. Coal miner's pneumoconiosis.
26. Phosgene poisoning.
27. Occupational cancer.
28. Isocyanides poisoning.
29. Toxic nephritis.

Asbestosis

Asbestosis is a chronic lung disease characterized by a scarring of lung tissues, which leads to long-term breathing complications. The disease does not have a cure.

Occupations with a high risk of asbestos exposure include

- Asbestos mining
- Asbestos plant workers
- Boiler workers

- Construction workers
- Fire-fighters
- Industrial workers
- Insulators
- Factory workers
- Power plant workers
- Shipyard workers
- Textile mill workers

Symptoms can include

- Coughing
- Chest pain
- Blood in the sputum
- Swelling in the neck or face
- Difficulty swallowing
- Loss of appetite
- Weight loss

How Is It Diagnosed?

Recommended diagnostic tools include:

- Complete physical examination
- Chest X-ray
- Lung function tests

A **lung biopsy**, in which tissue is removed by surgery, is the most reliable way to confirm the presence of microscopic asbestos fibers because X-rays cannot detect them.

Prevention

- Ensure that exposure to asbestos is kept as low as possible.
- If you have any concerns, stop work and talk to your supervisor.
- Don't eat, smoke or drink in the work area.
- Use personal protection; ensure it is clean and in good working order.
- Make sure the work area is clean at the end of the job.

Byssinosis

Byssinosis (brown lung disease) is a rare lung disease. It is caused by inhaling hemp, flax, and cotton particles. It is sometimes referred to as brown lung disease. It is a form of occupational asthma.

Causes of Byssinosis

Byssinosis is most common in textile industry workers. It is caused by inhalation of raw flax, hemp, cotton dust, and similar materials.

Smoking may increase the risk of developing byssinosis. A history of asthma or allergies may also increase risk.

Symptoms of Byssinosis

Symptoms of byssinosis usually appear during the beginning of the work week. They typically wane by the end of the week. If you are exposed to dust particles for long periods of time, you may experience symptoms during the entire week.

Symptoms of byssinosis

- Tightness in the chest
- Wheezing
- Coughing

Diagnosing Byssinosis

To diagnose byssinosis, doctor will ask questions about recent activities and work history

- Perform a physical exam to check your lungs.
- Chest X-rays and CT scans of lungs
- A peak flow meter tests how quickly you can expel air from your lungs

Prevention

Byssinosis is preventable.

If you work in a position that puts you at risk, wear a respiratory mask while working or near dust.

Lead Poisoning

Lead poisoning is a serious and sometimes fatal condition. It occurs when lead builds up in the body. Lead is a highly toxic metal and a very strong poison. It is found in lead-based paints; including paint on the walls of old houses and toys. It is also found in

- art supplies
- contaminated dust
- gasoline products
- Lead poisoning usually occurs over a period of months or years. The poisoning can cause severe mental and physical impairment.
- Severe lead poisoning is treated with chelation therapy and EDTA. However, damage from lead poisoning cannot be reversed.

What Causes Lead Poisoning?

Lead poisoning occurs when lead is ingested. It can also be caused by breathing in dust that contains lead. You cannot smell or taste lead. It is not visible to the naked eye.

Common sources of lead include

- pipes and sink faucets, which can contaminate drinking water
- storage batteries
- bullets, curtain weights, and fishing sinkers made of lead
- soil polluted by car exhaust or chipping house paint
- paint sets and art supplies

Who is at Risk for Lead Poisoning?

Children are at the highest risk of lead poisoning. There is a particularly high risk for children living in old houses with chipping paint. This is because children are prone to putting objects and fingers inside their mouths.

People in developing countries are also at a higher risk. Their countries do not have strict rules regarding lead. If you adopt a child from a developing country, his or her lead levels should be checked.

Symptoms of Lead Poisoning

Symptoms of lead poisoning are varied. They may affect many parts of the body. Most of the time, lead poisoning builds up slowly. It follows repeated exposures to small quantities of lead.

Lead toxicity is rare after a single exposure or ingestion of lead.

Signs of repeated lead exposure include:

- abdominal pain
- abdominal cramps
- constipation
- sleep problems
- headaches
- high blood pressure
- numbness or tingling in the extremities
- memory loss
- anaemia
- kidney dysfunction
- muscle weakness
- stumbling when walking

A high, toxic dose of lead poisoning may result in emergency symptoms.

Lead Poisoning Diagnosis

Lead poisoning is diagnosed with a blood lead test. This test is performed on a standard blood sample.

The amount of lead in the blood is measured in micrograms per decilitre (mcg/dL).

For adults, a normal result is less than 20 mcg/dL. Blood lead level greater than 60 mcg/dL is serious.

For children, a normal result is less than 10 mcg/dL, Blood lead level greater than 35-50mcg/dL is serious

Lead Poisoning Prevention

Simple steps can help you prevent lead poisoning. Some tips include

Avoid or throw away painted toys and canned goods from foreign countries.

- Keep your home free from dust.
- Use only cold water to prepare foods and drinks.
- Make sure everyone washes their hands before eating.
- Test your water for lead. If lead levels are high, consider using a filtering device. You can also drink bottled water.
- Clean faucets and aerators regularly.
- Wash children's toys and bottles regularly.
- Teach your children to wash their hands after playing.
- Make sure any contractor doing work in your house is certified in lead control.
- Use lead-free paint in your homes.
- Screen young children for blood lead levels.
- Avoid areas where lead based paint may have been used

Diagnosis methods of occupational diseases

Occupational disease is under-recognized. Failing to consider the workplace factors that may contribute to a patient's condition can result in the ordering of unnecessary tests, inappropriate referrals, and of equal or greater importance, a missed opportunity to protect others who may be at risk.

Clinical approach (personal)

- Clinical diagnosis
- Occupational exposure be observed
- Relationship between exposure and disease/symptoms
- High degree of exposure
- The Other factor of non-working
- The role of individual factor
- Occupational disease diagnose or not

Clinical Approach

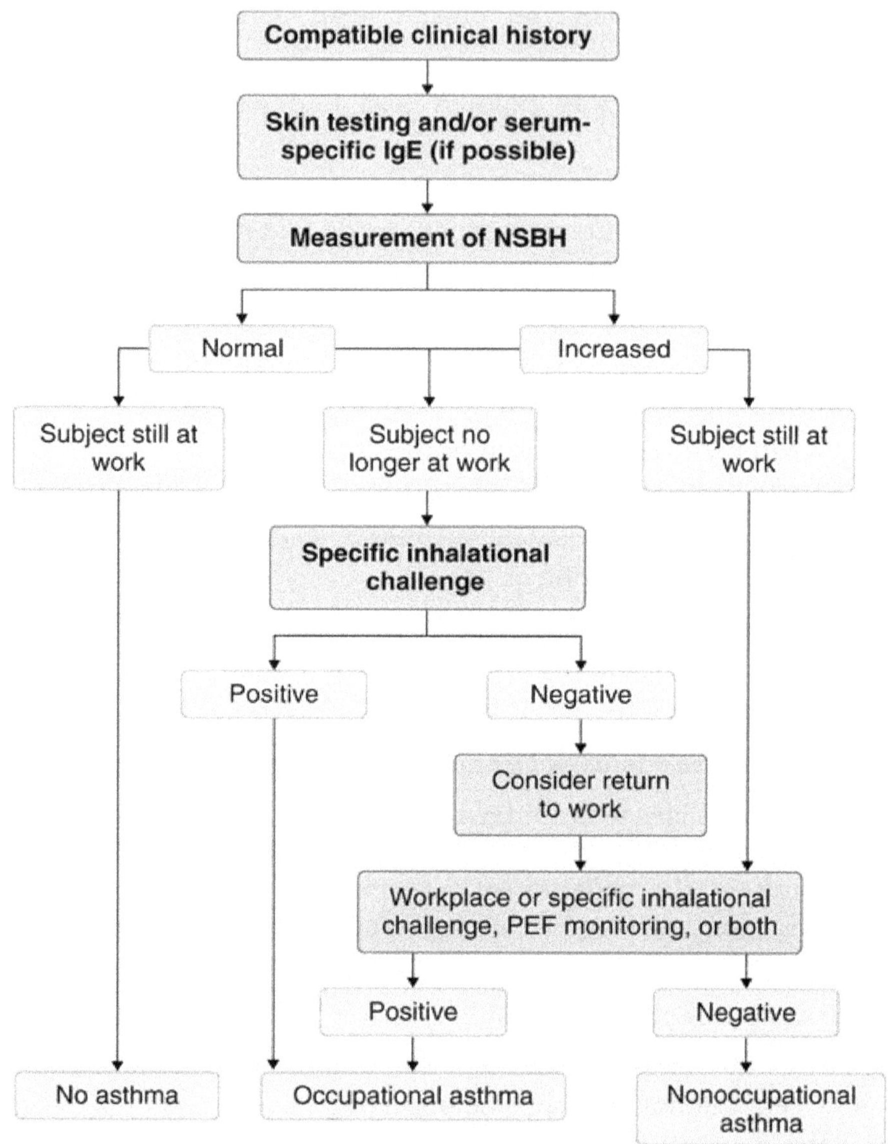

Silicosis

Silicosis is a chronic lung disease caused by breathing in tiny bits of silica dust. Silica is the second most common mineral in the earth's crust. It is a major component of sand, rock, and mineral ores like quartz.

Occupations leads to Silicosis

People who work in jobs where they are exposed to silica dust are at risk. These jobs include:

- Abrasives manufacturing
- Glass manufacturing
- Mining
- Quarrying
- Road and building construction
- Sand blasting
- Stone cutting

Symptoms of silicosis

Symptoms of silicosis may first appear 10-15 years after someone's exposure to crystalline silica. As the disease progresses, symptoms may include:

- Shortness of breath
- Severe cough
- Weakness

If you have silica in your lungs, your body may not be able to fight infections well. This can lead to other illnesses that can cause:

- Fever
- Weight loss
- Night sweats
- Chest pains
- Respiratory failure

As the disease progresses over time, these symptoms can become worse.

Silicosis diagnose

- Medical history including many questions about your current and past jobs, hobbies, and other activities through which you may have been exposed to silica
- Periodical physical exam

Prevention

The best way to prevent silicosis is to identify work-place activities that produce reparable crystalline silica dust and then to eliminate or control the dust ("primary prevention"). Water spray is often used where dust emanates. Dust can also be controlled through dry air filtering, Use respiratory protection.

Coal Worker's Pneumoconiosis

Coal worker's pneumoconiosis (CWP), also known as black lung disease or black lung, is caused by long exposure to coal dust. It is a common in coal miners and others who work with coal.

Types of Coal Worker's Pneumoconiosis

There are two types of coal worker's pneumoconiosis, simple coal worker's pneumoconiosis and progressive massive fibrosis (PMF) sometimes known as complicated coal worker's pneumoconiosis.

Simple coal worker's pneumoconiosis

Simple pneumoconiosis is the disease in its early form and is characterized by the presence of nodular aggregations within the lungs that occur at the site at which the coal dust has aggregated. A chest x-ray will determine the extent and severity of the disease. This form of the disease is asymptomatic and a fairly mild form. Many urban dwellers will unwittingly be sufferers due to poor air quality issues in some large cities.

Progressive massive fibrosis

The simple form of the disease can develop into progressive massive fibrosis if prolonged exposure to the source of dust is continued over time. PMF sufferers will develop large masses of dense fibrosis in the lungs which will lead to a decrease in lung function. It has been known for people suffering from PMF to be more susceptible to autoimmune conditions such as rheumatoid arthritis and scleroderma.

Symptoms

- Simple coal worker's pneumoconiosis
- Shortness of breath
- Chronic cough (with increased risk of chronic bronchitis)
- Progressive massive fibrosis:
- Shortness of breath
- Chronic cough

- Black sputum
- Lung dysfunction
- Pulmonary hypertension
- Heart problems
- There is no specific treatment for either simple coal worker's pneumoconiosis or complicated coal worker's pneumoconiosis.

Prevention

- Any worker that is in contact with dust that is known to cause pneumoconiosis conditions should be given a well-fitting facemask...
- Workers should be made aware of safe procedures with regard to the washing down of dust laden areas and of the removal and washing of clothes that have been exposed to the dust.
- Any part of the body exposed should be cleaned thoroughly and the worker should be mindful that dust should not be transmitted into the mouth by e.g. dust contaminated food, smoking, drinking, taking medicine, etc.

6.3 Biological Monitoring

Basic Concepts and Definitions

At the worksite, industrial hygiene methodologies can measure and control only airborne chemicals, while other aspects of the problem of possible harmful agents in the environment of workers, such as skin absorption, ingestion, and non-work-related exposure, remain undetected and therefore uncontrolled. Biological monitoring helps fill this gap.

Biological monitoring was defined in a 1980 seminar, jointly sponsored by the European Economic Community (EEC), National Institute for Occupational Safety and Health (NIOSH) and Occupational Safety and Health Association (OSHA) (Berlin, Yodaiken and Henman 1984) in Luxembourg as he measurement and assessment of agents or their metabolites either in tissues, secreta, excreta, expired air or any combination of these to evaluate exposure and health risk compared to an appropriate reference. Monitoring is a repetitive, regular and preventive activity designed to lead, if necessary, to corrective actions; it should not be confused with diagnostic procedures.

Biological monitoring is one of the three important tools in the prevention of diseases due to toxic agents in the general or occupational environment, the other two being environmental monitoring and health surveillance.

The sequence in the possible development of such disease may be schematically represented as follows: source-exposed chemical agent—internal dose—biochemical or cellular effect (reversible) —health effects—disease. The relationships among environmental, biological, and exposure monitoring, and health surveillance, are shown in figure.

When a toxic substance (an industrial chemical, for example) is present in the environment, it contaminates air, water, food, or surfaces in contact with the skin; the amount of toxic agent in these media is evaluated via environmental monitoring.

As a result of absorption, distribution, metabolism, and excretion, a certain internal dose of the toxic agent (the net amount of a pollutant absorbed in or passed through the organism over a specific time interval) is effectively delivered to the body, and becomes detectable in body fluids. As a result of its interaction with a receptor in the critical organ (the organ which, under specific conditions of exposure, exhibits the first or the most important adverse effect), biochemical and cellular events occur. Both the internal dose and the elicited biochemical and cellular effects may be measured through biological monitoring.

Health surveillance was defined at the above-mentioned 1980 EEC/NIOSH/OSHA seminar as his periodic medico-physiological examination of exposed workers with the objective of protecting health and preventing disease.

Biological monitoring and health surveillance are parts of a continuum that can range from the measurement of agents or their metabolites in the body via evaluation of biochemical and cellular effects, to the detection of signs of early reversible impairment of the critical organ. The detection of established disease is outside the scope of these evaluations.

Goals of Biological Monitoring

Biological monitoring can be divided into (a) monitoring of exposure, and (b) monitoring of effect, for which indicators of internal dose and of effect are used respectively.

The purpose of biological monitoring of exposure is to assess health risk through the evaluation of internal dose, achieving an estimate of the biologically active body burden of the chemical in question. Its rationale is to ensure that worker exposure does not reach levels capable of eliciting adverse effects. An effect is termed divers if there is an impairment of functional capacity, a decreased ability to compensate for additional stress, a decreased ability to maintain homeostasis (a stable state of equilibrium), or an enhanced susceptibility to other environmental influences.

Depending on the chemical and the analysed biological parameter, the term internal dose may have different meanings (Bernard and Lauwerys 1987). First, it may mean the amount of a chemical recently absorbed, for example, during a single work shift. A determination of the pollutant concentration in alveolar air or in the blood may be made during the work shift itself, or as late as the next day (samples of blood or alveolar air may be taken up to 16 hours after the end of the exposure period). Second, in the case that the chemical has a long biological half-life—for example, metals in the bloodstream—the internal dose could reflect the amount absorbed over a period of a few months.

Third, the term may also mean the amount of chemical stored. In this case it represents an indicator of accumulation which can provide an estimate of the concentration of the chemical in organs and/or tissues from which, once deposited, it is only slowly released. For example, measurements of DDT or PCB in blood could provide such an estimate.

Finally, an internal dose value may indicate the quantity of the chemical at the site where it exerts its effects, thus providing information about the biologically effective dose. One of the most promising and important uses of this capability, for example, is the determination of adducts formed by toxic chemicals with protein in haemoglobin or with DNA.

Biological monitoring of effects is aimed at identifying early and reversible alterations which develop in the critical organ, and which, at the same time, can identify individuals with signs of adverse health effects. In this sense, biological monitoring of effects represents the principal tool for the health surveillance of workers.

Principal Monitoring Methods

Biological monitoring of exposure is based on the determination of indicators of internal dose by measuring:

- The amount of the chemical, to which the worker is exposed, in blood or urine (rarely in milk, saliva, or fat)
- The amount of one or more metabolites of the chemical involved in the same body fluids
- The concentration of volatile organic compounds (solvents) in alveolar air
- The biologically effective dose of compounds which have formed adducts to DNA or other large molecules and which thus have a potential genotoxic effect.

Factors affecting the concentration of the chemical and its metabolites in blood or urine will be discussed below.

As far as the concentration in alveolar air is concerned, besides the level of environmental exposure, the most important factors involved are solubility and metabolism of the inhaled substance, alveolar ventilation, cardiac output, and length of exposure (Brugnone et al. 1980).

The use of DNA and haemoglobin adducts in monitoring human exposure to substances with carcinogenic potential is a very promising technique for measurement of low level exposures. (It should be noted, however, that not all chemicals that bind to macromolecules in the human organism are genotoxic, i.e., potentially carcinogenic.) Adduct formation is only one step in the complex process of carcinogenesis. Other cellular events, such as DNA repair promotion and progression undoubtedly modify the risk of developing a disease such as cancer. Thus, at the present time, the measurement of adducts should be seen as being confined only to monitoring exposure to chemicals. This is discussed more fully in the article enotoxic chemicals later in this chapter.

Biological monitoring of effects is performed through the determination of indicators of effect, that is, those that can identify early and reversible alterations. This approach may provide an indirect estimate of the amount of chemical bound to the sites of action and offers the possibility of assessing functional alterations in the critical organ in an early phase.

Advantages and Limitations of Biological Monitoring

For substances that exert their toxicity after entering the human organism, biological monitoring provides a more focused and targeted assessment of health risk than does environmental monitoring. A biological parameter reflecting the internal dose brings us one step closer to **Understanding systemic adverse effects than does any environmental measurement**

Biological monitoring offers numerous advantages over environmental monitoring and in particular permits assessment of:

- Exposure over an extended time period
- Exposure as a result of worker mobility in the working environment
- Absorption of a substance via various routes, including the skin
- Overall exposure as a result of different sources of pollution, both occupational and non-occupational
- The quantity of a substance absorbed by the subject depending on factors other than the degree of exposure, such as the physical effort required by the job, ventilation, or climate
- The quantity of a substance absorbed by a subject depending on individual factors that can influence the toxic kinetics of the toxic agent in the organism; for example, age, sex, genetic features, or functional state of the organs where the toxic substance undergoes biotransformation and elimination.

Biological gradient

The greater the level and duration of exposure, the greater the severity of diseases or their incidence.

Biological plausibility

From what is known of toxicology, chemistry, physical properties or other attributes of the studied risk or hazard, it makes biological sense to suggest that exposure leads to the disease.

Coherence

A general synthesis of all the evidence (e.g. human epidemiology and animal studies) leads to the conclusion that there is a cause–effect relationship in abroad sense and in terms of general common sense.

Interventional studies

Sometimes, a primary preventative trial may verify whether removing a specific hazard or reducing a specific risk from the working environment or work activity eliminates the development of a specific disease or reduces its incidence.

Criteria for identification and recognition of an individual disease

1. The exposure–effect relationship (relation between exposure and the severity of the impairment in the subject) and the exposure–response relationship (connection between exposure and the relative number of subjects affected) are important elements for the determination of a causal relationship. Research and epidemiological studies have greatly contributed in this respect. Better knowledge of the causal relationship has allowed us to achieve a better medical definition of occupational diseases. As a consequence, the legal definition of occupational diseases, which was rather a complex problem, is becoming more and more linked to the medical definition and criteria.
2. Legal provisions on compensation for victims vary from country to country. Article 8 of the Employment Injury Benefits Convention, 1964 [Schedule I amended in 1980] (No. 121), which indicates the various possibilities regarding the form of the identification and recognition of occupational diseases entitling.

6.3.1 Methods of Prevention of Occupational Disease

Good job safety and prevention practice can reduce your risk of occupational diseases try to stay fit, reduce stress, set up your work area properly and use the right protective equipment (PPE). An understanding of basic workplace health and safety issues means you can protect yourself against workplace hazards.

Recognize Risks/ Hazards or Safety Problems

There are some of the ways you can identify health and safety problems: observe your workplace

- Investigate complaints from workers
- Examine accident and near-miss records
- Examine sickness figures
- Use simple surveys to ask your co-workers about their health concerns
- Learn the results of inspections that are done
- Make sure you know and understand the hazards you are exposed to.
- Once you recognize a hazard, then you can determine which measure will correct the problem most effectively

Control measures

There are five major categories of control measures: elimination, Substitution, engineering controls, administrative controls & personal protective equipment

Eliminating or reducing exposure to the hazards in the workplaces

Eliminating a hazard means removing it completely; substitution is replacing one hazardous agent or work process with a less dangerous one. Elimination of a specific hazard or hazardous work process, or preventing it from entering the workplace, is the most effective method of control. If you cannot completely eliminate a hazard, then use a combination of control methods to protect yourself and your co-workers from being exposed to occupational hazards.

Changing Practices

When the existing ones are dangerous for the health (technical, engineering re-design, engineering control, administrative controls etc.). Engineering control may mean changing a piece of machinery (e.g., using proper machine guards) Administrative control for example is job rotation leading to working a limited number of hours in a hazardous area or changing a work process to reduce exposure to a hazard

Using adequate PPE

Including ear and eye protection, masks, respirators, and protective clothing – according to the exposure type.

Occupational Medical Screening

Occupational medical screening is intended to detect adverse health conditions that result from hazards and diagnose diseases existing in or derived from the workplace. The most effective control of occupational disease is by PRIMARY PREVENTION, which means preventing exposure or diminishing exposure to an acceptable level Secondary prevention or treatment of the exposed is less effective in reducing disease.

Screening programs are intended to supplement control efforts, not replace them the importance of screening is that it contributes to the early detection of disease in the individual and can lead to better prevention to those who share his exposures and risks.

Medical observation of individuals will highlight the hazards that are not controlled sufficiently, that way, health & safety policies can be improved in the company.

Personal hygiene (cleanliness)

Personal hygiene is also very important as a method of controlling hazards. Washing hands regularly, eating and smoking away from your work area help to prevent ingesting contaminants.

Your family can be exposed to the hazards you work with if you bring chemicals and other workplace contaminants home with you on your clothes, hair or skin. Before you leave work, wash/shower and change your clothes when necessary to prevent bringing workplace contaminants home.

Leave your dirty clothes at work or, if you must wash them at home, wash them separately, not with the family wash.

General measures

Think positive, try to solve the problems and responsibilities on time, have a healthy life style (including healthy foods, correct water intake of 2 liters of water/day, regular physical exercises, minimum eight sleeping hours daily) and try to create a positive atmosphere, not only in the workplace but also in the rest of your life in order to avoid supplementary problems.

Try to create a balance between work and family life, social life, do not overload yourself, divide projects into smaller phases, and prioritize tasks, delegate responsibilities to colleagues working with you in certain projects.

Always maintain a sense of humor, make sure to take short breaks throughout the day, to sit back and clear your mind.

Also try to get away from your desk for lunch. Stepping away from work to briefly relax and recharge will help you be more, not less, productive. Meditation, listening to music, walking for 5 minutes can improve your mood significantly.

Do not try to control the uncontrollable situations, adjust your standards, and be realistic about what you can accomplish.

6.4 Compensation for Occupational Diseases

General criteria for identification and recognition of occupational diseases:

1. The causal relationship is established on the basis of clinical and pathological data, Occupational background and job analysis, identification and evaluation of occupational risk factors and of the role of other risk factors.
2. Epidemiological and toxicological data are useful for determining the causal relationship between a specific occupational disease and its corresponding exposure in a specific working environment or work activity.
3. As a general rule, the symptoms are not sufficiently characteristic to enable an occupational disease to be diagnosed as such without the knowledge of the pathological changes engendered by the physical, chemical, biological or other factors encountered in the exercise of an occupation.
4. It is therefore normal that, as a result of improvements in knowledge regarding the mechanisms of action of the factors in question, the steady increase in the number of substances employed, and the quality and variety of suspected agents, it becomes more and more feasible to make an accurate diagnosis, while the range of diseases recognized as occupational in origin is broadening.

5. The recognition of a disease as being occupational is a specific example of clinical decision-making or applied clinical epidemiology.

Specificity

Exposure to a specific risk factor results in a clearly defined pattern of disease or diseases temporality or time sequence. The exposure of interest preceded the disease by a period of time consistent with any proposed biological mechanism.

Workers compensation benefits, states that:

Each Member shall:

(a) Prescribe a list of diseases, comprising at least the diseases enumerated in Schedule I to this Convention, which shall be regarded as occupational diseases under prescribed conditions;

(b) Include in its legislation a general definition of occupational diseases broad enough to cover at least the diseases enumerated in Schedule I to this Convention

(c) Prescribe a list of diseases in conformity with clause (a), complemented by a general definition of occupational diseases or by other provisions for establishing the occupational origin of diseases not so listed or manifesting themselves under conditions different from those prescribed.

1. Point (a) Is called the "list system",
   (b) Is the "general definition system" or overall coverage system
   (c) Is generally referred to as the "mixed system"
2. The "list system" covers only a certain number of occupational diseases, and has the advantage of listing diseases for which there is a presumption that they are of occupational origin. This simplifies the matter for all parties since it is frequently very difficult, if not impossible, to prove or disprove that a disease is directly attributable to the victim's occupation. It also has the important advantage of indicating clearly where prevention should focus.
3. The "general definition system" theoretically covers all occupational diseases; it affords the widest and most flexible protection, but leaves it to the victim to prove the

occupational origin of the disease. In practice, it also often implies that arbitration on individual cases is necessary. Furthermore, no emphasis is placed on specific prevention.

4. Because of this marked difference between the "general definition" and "list" systems, the "mixed system" has been favoured by many ILO member States because it combines the advantages of the other two without their disadvantages.

Biological monitoring of Occupational diseases

Biological monitoring is the measurement and assessment of chemicals or their metabolites (substances the body converts the chemical into) in exposed workers. These measurements are made on samples of breath, urine or blood, or any combination of these. Biological monitoring measurements reflect the total uptake of a chemical by an individual by all routes (inhalation, ingestion, through the skin or by a combination of these routes). Thus it differs from environmental monitoring which measures an individual's exposure. Biological monitoring of exposure is based on the determination of indicators of internal dose by measuring:

- The amount of the chemical, to which the worker is exposed, in blood or urine (rarely in milk, saliva, or fat)
- The amount of one or more metabolites of the chemical involved in the same body fluids
- The concentration of volatile organic compounds (solvents) in alveolar air
- The biologically effective dose of compounds which have formed adducts to DNA or other large molecules and which thus have a potential nontoxic effect.
- Exposure over an extended time period
- Exposure as a result of worker mobility in the working environment
- Absorption of a substance via various routes, including the skin
- Overall exposure as a result of different sources of pollution, both occupational and non-occupational
- The quantity of a substance absorbed by the subject depending on factors other than the degree of exposure, such as the physical effort required by the job, ventilation, or climate

- The quantity of a substance absorbed by a subject depending on individual factors that can influence the toxic kinetics of the toxic agent in the organism; for example, age, sex, genetic features, or functional state of the organs where the toxic substance undergoes biotransformation and elimination
- Knowledge of the metabolism of an exogenous substance in the human organism (toxic kinetics)
- Knowledge of the alterations that occur in the critical organ (toxic dynamics)
- Existence of sufficiently accurate analytical methods
- Possibility of using readily obtainable biological samples on which the indicators can be measured
- Existence of dose-effect and dose-response relationships and knowledge of these relationships
- Predictive validity of the indicators
- Existence of indicators
- The significance of biological indicators has not been clearly defined; for example, it is not always known whether the levels of a substance measured on biological material reflect current or cumulative exposure (e.g., urinary cadmium and mercury).

Occupational diseases are illnesses caused by substances or conditions that the employee was exposed to at the workplace. Schedule 3 of the Compensation for Occupational Injuries and Diseases Act sets out the working conditions and diseases caused by these conditions that are covered by the Compensation Fund. An employee can claim compensation if exposed to these working conditions and then getting the related disease. If a disease is not listed then employees can claim compensation only if they can prove that the disease was caused by conditions at work and not by some other factor. Medical evidence and reports will have to be submitted to the Commissioner. It may also take some time for a disease to become obvious and in such cases employees can claim compensation if they are no longer at a workplace so long as it falls within the time limits for lodging claims.

The Commissioner will approve or reject the claim. Only if the Commissioner approves the claim, will you get compensation (for temporary or permanent disability) and your medical expenses will be paid. If the disease gets worse after a period of time, you can apply to have your compensation increased.

6.5 Evaluation of Injuries

Injuries covered by the Compensation Act are only those that occur as a result of or at work. Compensation is paid for temporary and permanent disabilities that lead to a loss of earnings.

Types of compensation payment

Compensation is paid for getting injured at work or for diseases caused by work. There are four main types of compensation payments. These are:

- for temporary disability (the employee eventually recovers from the injury or illness)
- for permanent disability (the employee never fully recovers)
- for death
- for medical expenses
- additional compensation

Compensation is always worked out as a percentage of the wage the worker was earning at the time the disease or injury is diagnosed. If the worker is unemployed by the time a disease is diagnosed the wage they would have been earning must be calculated.

The Compensation Fund does not pay for pain and suffering, only for loss of movement or use of your body.

Temporary disability

Temporary disability means the employee does eventually get better. If an employee is off work for 3 days or less, no compensation will be paid (the employee can claim sick leave from the employer). If the employee is off for more than 3 days, the employee gets compensation which also covers the first 3 days. Temporary disability can be total or partial:

- Total means the employee is unable to work for a while. The employee will get % (75%) of the normal monthly wage as compensation. The formula is monthly wage x 75 ÷ 100, if the employee is paid monthly (for weekly paid employees, multiply the weekly wage by 4.3 to get the monthly wage)

- Partial means the employee can go to work, but on light duty for fewer hours. If the employee earns less doing the lighter work, he or she will get % of the difference between the normal and reduced monthly wage.

For an occupational disease, use the wage at the time of the diagnosis and not at the time when the employee first got exposed to the disease. If the employee is now unemployed, use the wage that he or she would probably have earned if still employed. Compensation for temporary disability will be paid for up to 12 months. If the condition of the employee has not improved after 12 months, the Commissioner may agree to continue payments for up to 24 months. After 24 months the Commissioner may decide that the condition is permanent and grant compensation on the basis of permanent disability. The Commissioner also pays all medical accounts, including medicine for which accounts must be submitted.

Permanent disability

Permanent disability means that an employee never fully recovers from the injury or sickness. A permanent disability can completely prevent an employee from working, or it can just inconvenience an employee. Most serious is called 100% disability, and least serious is called 1% disability. A doctor must write a medical report about the disability. The Commissioner, with the help of a panel of doctors, works out the degree of disability. The degrees of disability are set out in Schedule 2 of the Compensation for Occupational Injuries and Diseases Act. Some examples are:

- loss of two limbs 100%
- total loss of sight 100%
- loss of hearing in both ears 50%
- loss of sight in one eye 30%
- loss of one whole big toe 7%
- loss of one other toe 1%

Compensation for permanent disability is paid either as a monthly pension or as a lump sum:

- if the injury is measured as more than 30%, the employee gets a pension
- if the injury is 30% or less, the employee gets a lump sum

  The formula for the monthly pension is:

  [Monthly wage × (75 ÷ 100)] × (percentage disability ÷ 100)

  This amount will be paid once a month for the rest of the worker's life.
- The formula for the lump sum is:

  (Monthly wage × 15) × (percentage disability ÷ 100)

  This amount will be paid once only and there will be no further payments.

Death benefits

Compensation can be claimed by the widow or dependents if an employee dies as a result of a work-related accident or disease.

Claimants for death benefits must submit certified copies of the following documents:

- marriage certificate or proof that the couple lived as husband and wife
- birth certificates or baptismal certificates of children (for proof of children)
- the death certificate
- declaration by the widow
- the employer's report of the accident or disease
- funeral accounts
- a special Compensation form must be filled in, that details your income and property

Who can claim Compensation when an employee dies in the course and scope of duty?

- The widower
- Lump sum payment: 2 x monthly pension of employee (the pension is the amount the employee would have been paid if he/she had been 100% disabled)
- monthly pension for life: 40% x monthly pension of employee, paid every month

- Each child under the age of 18 years (including illegitimate, adopted and step children) is entitled to:
- 20% x monthly pension of employee, paid every monthly until the child is 18 years old
- the pension can continue for longer if the child is mentally or physically handicapped
- Other dependants, if there is no widow/err or children (parents, sisters, brothers, half-sisters, etc.):
- full dependants: get the same as the widow
- partial dependants: get a lump sum that is worked out according to the degree of dependence
- The person who pays for the funeral expenses: gets paid expenses up to Rs11.155.

The total monthly pension per family cannot be more than the pension the deceased worker would have received if he/she was 100% disabled (i.e. 75% of the monthly wage).

Medical expenses

All the medical expenses of a worker will be paid for a maximum of two years from the date of the accident.

Additional compensation

If an employee is injured, dies or contracts an occupational disease because of the negligence of the employer, or a defect in machinery or equipment, the employee can get extra compensation for temporary or permanent disability. Any employee who is under 26 years old at the time of an injury or disease will get extra compensation.

An application for additional (increased) compensation must be made on a form W930 within 24 months of the injury, The Commissioner can extend the period if good reasons exist.

The compensation office waits until it has all the forms and only then does it pay.

Temporary disability

The compensation office sends the money to the employer who gives it to the employee.

Permanent Disability

Lump sum: The money is paid to the employer. If an employee is no longer working for the same employer, they must leave details of their address with the employer.

Pension: This is paid out monthly for the rest of a person's life. The disabled employee can decide where the compensation office must send the pension, for example to a bank account. Pensions are always back-paid to the date of the accident.

If employers do not send in the forms or the claims takes long, employees must contact the nearest labour office and report it.

6.6 Occupational Health Management Services at Work Place

Surveillance of Work Environment and Risk Assessment

The surveillance of the work environment is one of the key activities of Basic Occupational Health Services. It is carried out for the identification of hazardous exposures and other conditions of work, identification of exposed workers and assessment of the levels of exposures for various groups of workers. Surveillance surveys must include the assessment of

- Ergonomic factors which might affect worker's health.
- Conditions of occupational hygiene and factors such as physical, chemical, biological exposures which may generate risks to the health of workers
- Exposure of workers to adverse psychological factors and aspects of work organization
- Risk of occupational accidents and major hazards
- Collective and personal protective equipment
- Control systems designed to eliminate, prevent or reduce exposure

Information from surveillance of the work environment is combined with information from health surveillance, and other relevant available data are used for risk assessment. It includes

- Identification of individuals and groups with special vulnerabilities

- Analysis of how the hazard may affect the worker
- Evaluation of available hazard prevention and control measures
- Making conclusions and recommendations for the management and control of risks
- Documenting the findings of the assessment
- Periodic review and, if necessary, reassessment of risks
- The results of risk assessment must be documented
- Identification of workers or groups of workers exposed to specific hazards
- Identification of occupational health hazards

Health surveillance and health examinations

The surveillance of worker's health is made through various types of health examinations. The main purpose of health examinations is to assess the suitability of a worker to carry out certain jobs, to assess any health impairment which may be related to the exposure to harmful agents inherent in the work process and to identify cases of occupational diseases which may have resulted from exposures at work. The following types of health examinations are carried out either on the basis of regulations or as a part of good occupational health practice.

- Pre-assignment (pre-employment) health examinations
- Periodic health examinations
- Return to work health examinations
- General health examinations
- Health examinations at termination or after ending of service

Advice on preventive and control measures

Occupational health services should propose appropriate prevention and control measures for the elimination of hazardous exposures and for protecting workers' health. Control measures should be adequate to prevent unnecessary exposure during normal operating conditions, as well as during possible accidents and emergencies. Guidelines for preventive actions for management and control of health and safety hazards and risk.

- Control of hazards at the source

- Ventilation or control technology
- Dust control
- Ergonomic measures
- Use of personal protective equipment
- Regulation of thermal conditions

Health education and health promotion, and promotion of work ability

Information on identified workplace health hazards and risks must be communicated to the managers responsible for implementing prevention and control measures. To ensure proper understanding and use of information the employer is responsible for education of his or her workers on risks and hazards at work and on their avoidance, prevention and protection, as well as on safe working practices. Such information and education tasks are often delegated to occupational health experts. The information and education include the following aspects.

- The workers have a right to know and get continuously information and training on hazards related to their own work and the workplace.
- Confidential health information of an individual worker is subject to special legislation and practices and to informed consent.

CHAPTER 7

Occupational Health Hazard

Occupational health hazard is defined as a disease caused by environmental factors, the exposure to which is peculiar to a particular process, ride, or occupation, and to which an employee is not ordinarily subjected or exposed outside of or away from such employment. A working condition that can lead to illness or death. Often, people in jobs which poses a high level of risk are paid more than similar but less risky jobs to compensate for the danger involved.

Danger to health, limb or life that is inherent in, or is associated with, a particular occupation, industry, or work environment. Occupational hazards include risk of accident and of contracting occupational diseases.

7.1 Occupational Hazards

A worker may be exposed to five different types of hazards, depending upon his/her occupation:

Physical hazards

Chemical hazards

Biological hazards

Mechanical hazards

Psychosocial hazards

Physical Hazards

1. ***Heat and cold:*** In India, the most common physical hazard is heat. The direct effect of heat exposure are burns, heat exhaustion, heat stroke and heat cramps; the indirect effects are decreased efficiency, increased fatigue and enhanced accident rates. Many industries have local hot spots – ovens and furnaces, which radiate heat. Radiant heat is main

problem in foundry, glass and steel industries, while heat stagnation is the principle problem in jute and cotton textiles. High temperatures are also found in mines. Physical work under such condition is very stressful and impairs the health and efficiency of the workers. For gainful work involving sustained and repeated effort, a reasonable temperature must be maintained in each work room.

Important hazards associated with cold work are chilblains, erythocyanosis, immersion foot, and frostbite as a result of cutaneous vasoconstriction. General hypothermia is not unusual.

2. ***Light:*** The workers may be exposed to risk of poor illumination or excessive brightness. The acute effects of poor illumination are eye strain, headache, eye pain, and lachrymation, congestion around the cornea and eye fatigue. The chronic effects on health includes "miner's nystagmus". Exposure to excessive brightness or glare is associated with discomfort, annoyance and visual fatigue. Intense direct glare may also result in blurring of vision and leads to accidents. There should be sufficient and suitable lighting, natural or artificial, wherever persons are working.

3. ***Noise:*** Noise is a health hazard in many industries. The effects of noise are of two type:
   (i) Auditory effects- which consist of temporary and permanent hearing loss
   (ii) Non-auditory effect- which consist of nervousness, fatigue, interference with communication by speech, decreased efficiency and annoyance.

The degree of injury from exposure to noise depends upon a number of factors such as intensity and frequency range, duration of exposure and individual susceptibility.

4. ***Vibration:*** Vibration, especially in the frequency range 10 to 500 Hz. May be encountered in work with pneumatic tools such as drills and hammers. Vibration usually affects the hands and arms. After some month or years of exposure, the fine blood vessels of the fingers may become increasingly sensitive to spasm (white finger).exposure to vibration may also produce injuries of the joints, of the hands, elbows and shoulders.

5. ***Ultraviolet radiation:*** Occupational exposure to ultraviolet radiation occurs mainly in arc welding. Such radiation occurs mainly affects the eyes, causing intense conjunctivitis and keratitis (welder's flash). Symptoms are redness of eye and pain, these usually disappear in few days with no permanent effect on the vision or on the deeper structures of the eye.
6. ***Ionizing radiation:*** Ionizing radiation is finding increasing application in medicine and industry, e.g. x-rays and radioactive isotopes. Important radio isotopes are cobalt60 and phosphorus32. Certain tissues such as bone marrow are more sensitive than others and from a genetic standpoint, there are special hazards when the gonads are exposed. The radiation hazards comprise genetic changes, malformation, cancer, leukaemia, depilation, ulceration, sterility and in extreme cases death. The international commission of radiological protection has set the maximum permissible level of occupational exposure at 5 rem per year to the whole body.

Chemical Hazards

There is hardly any industry which does not make use of chemicals. The chemical hazards are on the increase with the introduction f newer and complex chemicals. Chemical agents act in three ways; local action, inhalation and ingestion. The ill-effects produced depend upon the duration of exposure, the quantum of exposure and individual susceptibility.

1. **Local action:** Some chemicals cause dermatitis, eczema, ulcers and even cancer by primary irritant action; some cause dermatitis by an allergic action. Some chemicals, particularly the aromatic nitro and amino compounds such as TNT and aniline are absorbed through the skin and cause systemic effects. Occupational dermatitis is a big problem in industry.
2. **Inhalation**
   (i) Dusts-dusts are finely divided solid particles with size ranging from 0.1 to 150 microns. They are released into the atmosphere during crushing, grinding, abrading, loading and unloading operation. Dusts are produced in a number of industries – mines, foundry quarry, pottery,

textile, wood or stone working industries. Dust particle larger than 10 microns settle done from the air rapidly, while the smaller ones remain suspended indefinitely. Particles smaller than 5 microns are directly inhaled into lungs and are retained there. This fraction of dust is called" respiratory dust", and is mainly responsible for pneumoconiosis. Dusts have been classified into inorganic and organic dusts; soluble and insoluble dusts. The inorganic dusts are silica, mica, coal, asbestos dust; etc. The organic dust are cotton, jute and the like. The soluble dusts remain, more or less, permanent in the lungs. They are mainly the cause of pneumoconiosis. The most common dust diseases are silicosis and anthracnoses.

(ii) Gases- exposure to gases is a common hazard in industries. Gases are sometimes classified as simple gases (e.g. oxygen, hydrogen), asphyxiating gases (e.g. carbon monoxide, cyanide gas, sulphur dioxide, chlorine) and aesthetic gases (e.g. chloroform, ether, and trichloroethylene). Carbon monoxide hazard is frequently reported in coal-gas manufacturing plants and steel industry.

(iii) Metal and their compounds- a large number of metals and their compounds are used throughout industry. The chief mode of entry of some of them is by inhalation as dust or fumes. The industrial physician should be aware of toxic effects of lead, antimony, arsenic, beryllium, cadmium, cobalt, manganese, mercury, phosphorus, chromium, zinc and others. The ill-effects depend upon the duration of exposure and the dose or concentration of exposure. Unlike the pneumoconiosis, most chemical intoxications respond favourably to cessation, exposure and medical treatment.

3. **Ingestion:** Occupational diseases may also result from ingestion of chemical substance such as lead, mercury, arsenic, zinc, chromium, cadmium, phosphorus, etc. Usually these substances are swallowed in minute amounts through contaminated hands, food or cigarettes. Much of the ingested material is excreted through faeces and only a small proportion may reach the general blood circulation.

Biological Hazards

Workers may be exposed to infective and parasitic agents at the place of work. The occupational diseases in this category are brucellosis, leptospirosis, anthrax, hydatidosis, psittacosis, tetanus, encephalitis, fungal infection, schistosomiasis and a host of others. Persons working among animal products (e.g. hair, wool, hides) and agricultural workers are specially exposed to biological hazards.

Mechanical Hazards

The mechanical hazards in industry centre round machinery, protruding and moving parts and the like. About 10% of accidents in industry are said to be due to mechanical causes.

Psychosocial Hazards

The psychosocial hazards arise from the workers failure to adapt to an alien psychosocial environment. Frustration, lack of job satisfaction, insecurity, poor human relationships, emotional tension are some of the psychosocial factors which may undermine both physical and mental health of the workers. The capacity to adapt to different working environment is influenced by many factors such as education, cultural background, family life, social habits and what the worker experts from employment.

The health effects can be classified in two main categories

(a) Psychological and behavioural changes – including hostility, aggressiveness, anxiety, depression, tardiness, alcoholism, drug abuse, sickness absenteeism.

(b) Psychosomatic illhealth – including fatigue, headache, pain in the shoulders, neck and back; propensity to pepyic ulcer, hypertension, heart disease and rapid aging.

The physical factors (heat, noise, poor lighting) play a major role in adding to or precipitating mental disorders among workers. The increasing stress on automation, electronic operations and nuclear energy may introduce newer psychosocial health problems in industry. Psychosocial hazards are these fore assuming more importance than physical or chemical hazards.

7.1.1 Adverse Health Effects from Noise

Noise health effects are the health consequences of regular exposure, to consistent elevated sound levels. Elevated workplace or other noise can cause hearing impairment, hypertension, ischemic heart disease, annoyance, and sleep disturbance.

Noise, defined as 'unwanted sound', is perceived as an environmental stressor and nuisance. Non-auditory effects of noise, as dealt with in this chapter, can be defined as 'all those effects on health and well-being which are caused by exposure to noise, with the exclusion of effects on the hearing organ and the effects which are due to the masking of auditory information.

Exposure to continuous noise of 85–90 dBA, particularly over a lifetime in industrial settings, can lead to a progressive loss of hearing, with an increase in the threshold of hearing sensitivity. Hearing impairments due to noise are a direct consequence of the effects of sound energy on the inner ear. However, the levels of environmental noise, as opposed to industrial noise, are much lower and effects on non-auditory health cannot be explained as a consequence of sound energy.

If noise does cause ill-health other than hearing impairment, what might be the mechanism?

It is generally believed that noise disturbs activities and communication, causing annoyance. In some cases, annoyance may lead to stress responses, then symptoms and possibly illness. Alternatively, noise may influence health directly and not through annoyance. The response to noise may depend on characteristics of the sound, including intensity, frequency, and complexity of sound, duration and the meaning of the noise.

Effects of Noise on Health

Health Effects

Exposure to high levels of noise can cause permanent hearing loss. Neither surgery nor a hearing aid can help correct this type of hearing loss. Short term exposure to loud noise can also cause a temporary change in hearing (your ears may feel stuffed up) or a ringing in your ears (tinnitus). These short-term problems may go away within a few minutes or hours after leaving the noise.

However, repeated exposures to loud noise can lead to permanent tinnitus and/or hearing loss.

Noise and sleep disturbance

There is both objective and subjective evidence for sleep disturbance by noise. Exposure to noise disturbs sleep proportional to the amount of noise experienced in terms of an increased rate of changes in sleep stages and in number of awakenings. Habituation occurs with an increased number of sound exposures by night and across nights. One laboratory study, however, found no habituation during 14 nights of exposure to noise at maximum noise level exposure. Objective sleep disturbance is likely to occur if there are more than 50 noise events per night with a maximum level of 50 dBA indoors or more. In fact, there is a low association between outdoor noise levels and sleep disturbance.

Noise exposure during sleep may increase blood pressure, heart rate and finger pulse amplitude as well as body movements. There may also be after-effects during the day following disturbed sleep; perceived sleep quality, mood and performance in terms of reaction time all decreased following sleep disturbed by

Noise exposure and performance

There is good evidence, largely from laboratory studies, that noise exposure impairs performance. Performance may be impaired if speech is played while a subject reads and remembers verbal material, although this effect is not found with non-speech noise. The effects of 'irrelevant speech' are independent of the intensity and meaning of the speech. The susceptibility of complex mental tasks to disruption by 'irrelevant speech' suggests that reading, with its reliance on memory, may also be impaired.

Perceived control over and predictability of noise has been found to be important in determining effects and after-effects of noise exposure. Glass and Singer found that tasks performed during noise were unimpaired but tasks that were carried out after noise had been switched off were impaired, this being reduced when subjects were given perceived control over the noise. Indeed, even anticipation of a loud noise exposure in the absence of real exposure may impair performance and an expectation of control counters this effect. Noise exposure may also slow rehearsal in memory, influence processes of selectivity in memory, and choice of strategies for carrying out tasks. There is also evidence that noise may reduce helping behaviour, increase aggression and reduce the processing of social cues seen as irrelevant to task performance.

Noise and Cardiovascular Disease

Physiological responses to noise exposure

Noise exposure causes a number of predictable short-term physiological responses mediated through the autonomic nervous system. Exposure to noise causes physiological activation including increase in heart rate and blood pressure, peripheral vasoconstriction and thus increased peripheral vascular resistance. There is rapid habituation to brief noise exposure but habituation to prolonged noise is less certain.

Occupational studies: noise and high blood pressure

The strongest evidence for the effect of noise on the cardiovascular system comes from studies of blood pressure in occupational settings. Many occupational studies have suggested that individuals chronically exposed to continuous noise at levels of at least 85 dB have higher blood pressure than those not exposed to noise. In many of these studies, noise exposure has also been an indicator of exposure to other factors, both physical and psychosocial, which are also associated with high blood pressure. Unless these other risk factors are controlled, spurious associations between noise and blood pressure may arise. A recent pioneering longitudinal industrial noise study has shown that noise levels predicted raised systolic and diastolic pressure in those doing complex but not simple jobs, and predicts increased mortality risk. Occupational noise exposure has also recently been linked to greater risk of death from motor vehicle injury. One possibility is that the effects of noise on blood pressure are mediated through an intermediate psychological response such as noise annoyance although this has not been convincingly proved.

7.1.2 Adverse Health Effects of Vibration

What are the health effects of hand-arm vibration?

Vibration induced health conditions progress slowly. In the beginning it starts as a pain. As the vibration exposure continues, the pain may develop into an injury or disease. Pain is the first health condition that is noticed and should be addressed in order to stop the injury.

Vibration-induced white finger (VWF) is the most common condition among the operators of hand-held vibrating tools. Vibration can cause changes in tendons, muscles, bones and joints, and can affect the nervous system. Collectively, these effects are known as Hand-Arm Vibration Syndrome (HAVS). The symptoms of VWF are aggravated when the hands are exposed to cold.

Workers affected by HAVS commonly report

- attacks of whitening (blanching) of one or more fingers when exposed to cold
- tingling and loss of sensation in the fingers
- loss of light touch
- pain and cold sensations between periodic white finger attacks
- loss of grip strength
- bone cysts in fingers and wrists

What are the symptoms of hand-arm vibration syndrome (HAVS)?

Hand-arm vibration exposure affects the blood flow (vascular effect) and causes loss of touch sensation (neurological effect) in fingers.

What are the health effects of whole-body vibration?

Whole-body vibration can cause fatigue, insomnia, stomach problems, headache and "shakiness" shortly after or during exposure. The symptoms are similar to those that many people experience after a long car or boat trip. After daily exposure over a number of years, whole-body vibration can affect the entire body and result in a number of health disorders. Sea, air or land vehicles cause motion sickness when the vibration exposure occurs in the 0.1 to 0.6 Hz frequency range. Studies of bus and truck drivers found that occupational exposure to whole-body vibration could have contributed to a number of circulatory, bowel, respiratory, muscular and back disorders. The combined effects of body posture, postural fatigue, dietary habits and whole-body vibration are the possible causes for these disorders.

Studies show that whole-body vibration can increase heart rate, oxygen uptake and respiratory rate, and can produce changes in blood and urine. East European researchers have noted that exposure to whole-body vibration can produce an overall ill feeling which they call "vibration sickness."

Many studies have reported decreased performance in workers exposed to whole-body vibration.

Factors that influence the effect of vibration on the hand		
Physical Factors	**Biodynamic Factors**	**Individual Factors**
Acceleration of vibration	Grip forces - how hard the worker grasps the vibrating equipment	Operator's control of tool
Frequency of vibration	Surface area, location, and mass of parts of the hand in contact with the source of vibration	Machine work rate
Duration of exposure each workday	Hardness of the material being contacted by the hand-held tools, for example metal in grinding and chipping	Skill and productivity
Years of employment involving vibration exposure	Position of the hand and arm relative to the body	Individual susceptibility to vibration
State of tool maintenance	Texture of handle-soft and compliant versus rigid material	Smoking and use of drugs. Exposure to other physical and chemical agents.
Protective practices and equipment including gloves, boots, work-rest periods.	Medical history of injury to fingers and hands, particularly frostbite	Disease or prior injury to the fingers or hands

Why is it not easy to diagnose vibration related diseases?

The acceptance of vibration syndrome as an industrial disease is hindered mainly because:

- Not every physician is trained to diagnose vibration-induced white finger (VWF) or other vibration-related diseases.
- The causes of VWF cannot always be identified.
- There are no objective clinical tests to measure the impairment.

7.1.3 Adverse Health Effects of Cold

Having a low temperature or inadequate temperature feeling or a sensation of coldness. Generally, in this low temperatures mortality increases. The prolonged action of this cold periods is well denoted to be as cold spells. Cold spells are defined to be as the event below the temperature threshold lasting for a minimum duration of two days.

A cold environment may cause several adverse effects on human functions (or) performance and it also effects on health. The cold exposure is mostly seen in Barnet's region and in this barent's region, there are various occupational activities. Where the employees who work in that region are frequently exposed to cold. And also this cold exposure is mostly seen in northern work places, so to avoid or control this cold exposure case, some new practical methods and principles of operation were produced related to cold risk assessment, management and occupational health care and this new practical's methods were tested only by the key persons of the target companies of the parent's region. The climates of Nordic countries are generally controlled by westerly air streams.

The lowest winter temperatures are generally occur in northern Finland and Sweden and in this parent's region the occupational distribution differ from country to country. In northern parts of Nordic countries different services for societies, infrastructure involve cold exposure well known fact that fisherman are mostly exposed to cold work exposure

There Isa evidence from epidemiological studies that human daily mortality mainly related to temperature during the day or preceding days. And there is also a small evidence that adverse effects of cold are more pronounced in warmer climates and vice versa and thus these effects are not probably not so much associated with universal temperature level as they are with a temperature level that is relative to the prevailing climate.

In addition to this effects of the level of the temperature per se, there is some evidence that a change in temperature over time could have adverse health effects .the effects of exposure to cold could be modified by the type of climate , season, housing conditions, or factors defining the susceptibility of the population exposed to cold spells.

Physiological and pathological effects of short term exposure to cold are known. Low atmospheric temperature induces vasoconstriction, increases systolic and diastolic blood pressure, blood viscosity, blood cholesterol in matter of hours which may increase the risk of myocardial infarction and stroke. Exposure to cool air also enhances diuresis.

The Effects of Cold on Human

The effects of cold on human are mainly dependent on the basic parameters of environmental factors such as temperature, wind, and humidity. And also depend upon the degree of activity such as light or heavy work and also the type of clothing used.

Depending up on the variations or interactions on these variables cold stress causing local or whole body cooling may occur. This cold stress affects the whole human body performance and may result in different effects from discomfort to cold injuries. The actual risk of these effects is largely dependent on individual factors.

Cold and Performance

Depending upon the level of local or whole body cooling different levels of performance degradation may occur.

The term “performance include physical such as example: muscular. And also manual and cognitive for example such as mental performance.

Mild cold stress causes thermal discomfort resulting in complaints of cold, unpleasantness and even pain. Discomfort may represent a distracting factor that can reduce mental alertness increasing the reaction times and also the amount of errors and also destroy the quality of work.

Under severe cold exposure even long term memory and consciousness may be effected and this cooling effects components of muscular performance, force, power and also the co-ordination and even a small mild level cooling of the muscles may mostly effect physical performance, this type of cooling may occur frequently when working in cold .

Cold decreases the manual performance in sever always and this may result in clumsiness and also the ability to perform fine movements of the hand and some people will experience pain.

And so this cold also affects the cognitive performance on human. More importantly the complex tasks which are performed in the cold are mainly susceptible to body cooling.

Symptoms and Cold Related Diseases

Cold exposure involve a variety of different complaints ranging from subjective uncomfortable sensations to symptoms related to diseases (H Cold related) diseases are defined as diseases which are either caused by cold or which symptoms are produced during cold exposure. Therefore, these include many of the most common chronic diseases like respiratory and cardiovascular diseases.

Certain individuals may also be especially susceptible to cold exposure. In these persons certain 'hyper reactions' to cold may occur. These include for example an exaggerated constriction of blood vessels in hands (Raynaud's phenomenon), internal organs such as kidney, lungs, heart, or eyes due to cold exposure.

These reactions may cause different types of functional disturbances of varying severity in human. Furthermore, persons having different cold symptoms are very sensitive to cold discomfort, too.

Cold Injuries

Recent studies have shown that Incidences of frostbites occur relatively frequently during occupational duties. Frostbites result often in different functional disadvantages, some of which can lead to a temporary or permanent disability to work. Different types of abnormalities are commonly associated with frostbite injuries. Further, frostbites cause often abnormality lasting from a few weeks to a lifetime.

Whole body cooling below body temperature 35°C is defined as hypothermia and is a type of cold injury. Severe whole body cooling occurs rarely in occupational situations.

Cold Associated Injuries

As a consequence of director in direct effects of cold, the total injury rate may be changed in relation to environmental conditions. It is worth noting that cold associated injuries are not always s caused purely due to alteration sin the work environment such as ice and snow. Body cooling may result in impaired performance, which may increase the risk for accidents. The unsafe behavior of workers seems to be minimal at an environmental temperature of +20° canda shift to cooler or warmer temperatures increases the risk for accidents.

Cold Related Diseases

- ***Respiratory:*** Asthma and infections
- ***Cardiovascular:*** Coronary and other heart disease, andmyo-cardial infarction
- ***Dermatological:*** Cold urticarial and psoriasis.
- Injuries, such as frostbite and trench foot.

Cold Related Deaths

Total higher mortality in most population is higher in win ter than in summer causes for death: coronary heart diseases and respiratory diseases.

Conclusion

Cold work involves several adverse effects that are observed both in outdoor and indoor work many of these adverse out comes may be further aggravated in persons have a chronic disease. For indoor work, the climatic conditions are conditions are constant and predict table, therefore health consequences related to working in cold climate will remain common mitigation of the adverse effects and adaptation to the climate change in cold outdoor work will require inter disciplinary analyses and integrated preventive planning.

The disease progresses for years before the symptoms become severe enough to affect a worker's ability to do her or his work.

7.1.4 Adverse Health Effects of Heat

The adverse health effects of hot weather and heat-waves are not easily preventable. Prevention requires a role of actions at different levels. These actions can be formed in a defined heat–health action plan. These high temperatures have health effects under all latitudes and on northern populations too, and Canadians are no exception. Various risk indicators associated with the adverse health impacts of heat in industrialized countries have been reported in the scientific literature, particularly since the European heat wave. Among these indicators, advancing age is well recorded, while low socio economic level appears to be strongly predictive of disease and poor quality of life. In Canada, poverty is mainly an urban problem. In fact, Canada's large urban regions and its metropolitan census regions have a disproportionate number of poor people. In addition, pockets of poverty are often concentrated in certain areas which generally correspond to the most socially and materially disadvantaged census dissemination areas. These areas present a group of factors strongly correlated with high heat and humidity discomfort, particularly in densely populated cities where the heat island effect extends over large areas and may reach a greater intensity as compared with rural or semi-urban regions.

Recommendation to the public during heat waves

Keep your home cool

Keep your living room cool and ideally the room temperature should be kept below 32°C during the day and 24°C during the night. This is especially important for infants or people who are over 60 years of age or have chronic health conditions.

Use the night air to cool down your home. Open all windows and shutters during the night and the early morning, when the outside temperature is lower.

Reduce the heat load inside the apartment or house. Close windows and shutter especially those facing sun during the day.

Hang wet towels to cool down the room air. Note that the humidity of the air increases at the same time.

If your residence is air conditioned, close the doors and windows and conserve electricity not needed to keep you cool, to ensure that power remains available and reduce the chance of a community-wide outage.

Keep out of heat

- Move to the coolest room in the home, especially at night.
- If it is not possible to keep your home cool, spend 2–3 hours of the day in a cool place
- Avoid going outside during the hottest time of the day
- Stay in the shade
- Do not leave children or animals in parked vehicles

- Keep the body cool and hydrated
- Take cool showers or baths. Alternatives include cold packs and wraps and towels
- Wear light, loose-fitting clothes of natural materials. If you go outside, wear a wide-brimmed hat or cap and sunglasses
- Use light bed linen and sheets, and no cushions, to avoid heat accumulation
- Drink regularly, but avoid alcohol and too much caffeine and sugar
- Help others
- Plan to check on family, friends, and neighbours who spend much of their time alone
- Discuss extreme heat-waves with your family. Everyone should know what to do in the places where they spend time
- If anyone you know is at risk. Help him or her to get advice and support. Elderly or sick people living alone should be visited at least daily
- If a person is taking medication, ask the treating doctor how it can influence thermoregulation and the fluid balance

If you have health problem

- Keep medicines below 25 °C or in the refrigerator (read the storage instructions on the packaging)
- Seek medical advice if you are suffering from a chronic medical condition

Risk Factors for Heat Illnesss and Mortality

In addition to the information for the general public, certain information should be provided for population groups at high risk of health effects from heat-waves. Elderly and very elderly people with chronic diseases

Practical tips (such as for keeping cool and well hydrated)

Information on first aid treatment.

Important contact details for social and medical services, including ambulance services.

Risk factors include

In elderly and very elderly people the changes is seen in thermo regulation and renal function and also health status.

In female and elderly and very elderly people the changes is seen in difference in thermo physiological functioning.

In infants changes is generally seen thermo regulation immature, smaller body mass, blood volume level dehydration risk in case of diarrhea.

Risk factors related to health

Acute health conditions: Conditions such as acute renal failure, cerebrovascular disease, heart failure, pneumonia and infectious diseases during heat waves.

Chronic health conditions: reduced thermoregulatory ability, high risk of acute events, exacerbations of disease, reduced ability to care for oneself, and take appropriate protective action and/or seek assistance Cardiovascular and respiratory diseases and their treatment are of highest priority.

Risk factors related to socio economic

Low economic status (poverty; low income), low educational level: Poor people tend to have a higher underlying prevalence of chronic diseases, lower housing quality and less well-heated and cooled homes.

Being homeless: Lack of shelter, concomitant chronic diseases (physical and psychiatric diseases)

Not leaving home daily: Lack of social interaction.

Lack of social interaction: Lack of advice on and treatment of existing health conditions, and delay in care for heat-related conditions.

Risk factors related to environment conditions

Air pollution: Combined effect of high temperature and air pollution.

Occupational exposures (especially for males): High exposure levels that reduce thermoregulatory ability, risk of dehydration.

Urban areas: Cities tend to become hotter than surrounding areas due to the heat is land effect. This increases the severe heat stress experienced during the day and further impairs the body tolerance of heat combined with the absence of relief at night.

Many chronic health conditions require medical treatment with drugs that in turn might raise the risk of health effects through heat exposure. Instead of adjusting essential medication, it is advisable to ensure that these patients have access to cool places and are not exposed to heat.

Conclusion

In conclusion, the present study documented the prevalence of reported health impacts during very hot and summer conditions in the most disadvantaged dissemination areas of most populated cities. Those under 65 years of age and in those 65 years of age and older. Female sex, long-term medical leave, and very low income suggest biological, or contextual differences that can have an impact either on heat exposure or on adaptation of both of the age groups. It appears that the scope of the indicators associated with the prevalence of health impacts should be broadened to other categories of variables, such as the characteristics of the dwelling and lifestyle

From existing community surveys and health surveillance reports. Relevant further research should focus on: (1) validity of self-reported heat exposure; (2) better identification of chronic diseases compromising thermoregulation; (3) better understanding of the mechanisms underlying the differences in sex-based health impacts in a context of heat; (4) better assessment of indoor temperature as an exposure variable for heat impacts.

7.1.5 Adverse Health Effects of Stress

Stress is the body's reaction to any change that requires an adjustment or response. The body reacts to these changes with physical, mental, and emotional responses.

Stress is a normal part of life. Many events that happen to you and around you -- and many things that you do yourself -- put stress on your body. You can experience stress from your environment, your body, and your thoughts.

The human body is designed to experience stress and react to it. Stress can be positive, keeping us alert and ready to avoid danger. Stress becomes negative when a person faces continuous challenges without relief or relaxation between challenges.

As a result, the person becomes overworked and stress-related tension builds.

Classification of stressors

Physical stressors: Extreme of temperature, lighting, ventilation, and humidity, noise and vibration.

Chemical stressors: Dangerous chemicals, gases, vapours, dusts...etc

Biological stressors: Bacteria, virus...etc

Effects of stress: Stresses vary considerably from person to person. Typical effects of stress are headaches, insomnia, fatigue, over eating, constipation, nervousness, minor accidents, palpitations, indigestion and irritability.

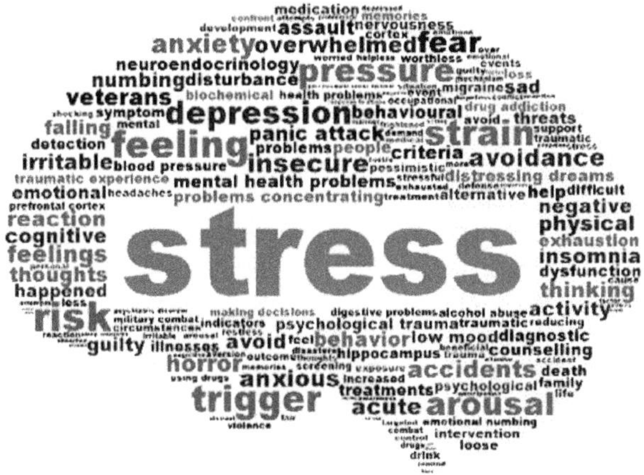

The two more principal psychological effects of stress are anxiety and depression.

1. **Anxiety:** This is a state of tension coupled with apprehension, worry, guilt, insecurity and a constant need for reassurance. It is accompanied by psychosomatic, symptoms such as profuse perspiration, difficulty in breathing, gastric disturbances, rapid heartbeat, frequent urination, muscle tension or high blood pressure. Insomnia is a reliable indicator of a state of anxiety.

2. **Depression:** this has been defined as 'a sadness which has lost its relationship to a logical progression of events'. another definition is 'a mood, characterized by feeling of dejection and gloom and other permutations, such as feeling of hopelessness, futility and guilt'

Typical stressful conditions

1. Too heavy or too light a work load.
2. A job which is too difficult or too easy.
3. Working excessive hours.
4. Conflicting the job demands.
5. Poor human relationship.
6. Lack of participation in decision.
7. Middle-age vulnerability associated with reduced career prospects.
8. Over-promotion or under-promotion.
9. Interaction between work and family commitments.

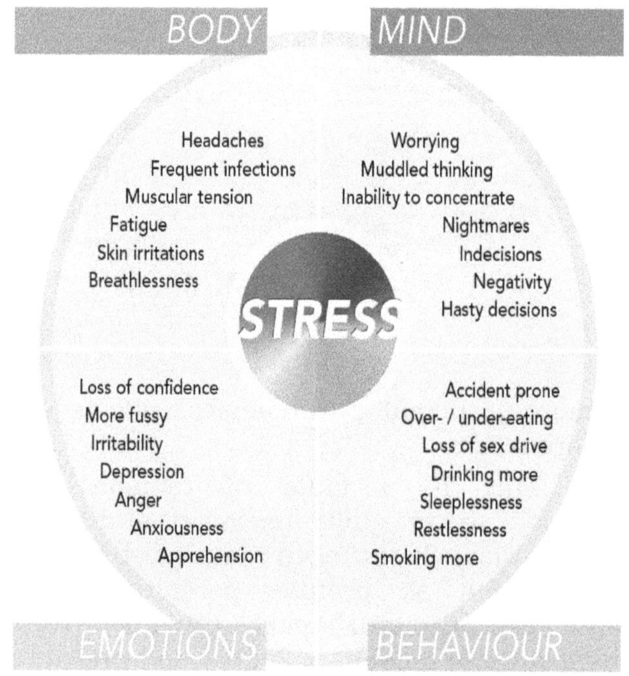

7.1.6 Adverse Health Effects of Improper Illumination

Light

The natural agent that stimulates sight and makes things visible. The word usually refers to visible light, which is visible to the human eye and is responsible for the sense of sight. Visible light is usually defined as having wavelength in the range of 400–700 nanometers (nm), between the infrared and the ultraviolet. This wavelength means a frequency range of roughly 430–750terahertz (THz). Often, infrared and ultraviolet are also called light.

The introduction of computers in the 1970's increased the visual demands of our work and made lighting design even more challenging. While typewriters were being exchanged for computers, the need for redesigning or rearranging office lighting was commonly overlooked.

Human Physiology

As for the eye, we know that light can produce both systemic physiologic responses and cognitive stimulate. For light to be perceived, it must traverse the optical pathway to the brain. This means that the eye itself must be optically clear, the retina healthy, the optic nerve intact, and the various parts of the brain responsible for light detection and vision, functional. For now, let's assume an operational visual pathway.

A. *Autonomous Physiologic Effects*: Research has shown conclusively that light affects the human body in ways other than producing vision. The effects identified so far involve body rhythms. There are currently over 3000 references on light's effect on human chronobiolog. We will look first at a controversial one.

B. Psychological Effects: Visible light, or the lack thereof, can affect our mood through neuron-physiology. Lighting can also affect our mood based on our cognitive perceptions, and possibly unconscious perceptions. Unfortunately, there has been very little research in this area. Studies of the effects of ambient colour used in indoor environments have been proposed, but rarely funded. There is anecdotal mention of the use of pink in jails to 'mellow out' prisoners, but there has been no real follow-up. This is a ripe area for study.

To further complicate matters, standard eyewear can actually exacerbate some problems. The most common lens is made of CR-39 plastic resin, which has a refractive index n = 1.50. At this index, only 92% of light will get to the eye, due to front and back-surface reflections. Inter-reflections can also produce significant levels of glare, especially at night. If polycarbonate is used (what the author wears) with n = 1.585, or the newer high-index resins (n = 1.59 +), the light loss is greater, and glare worse. A solution will be mentioned later.

Complaints and Fears

1. *Eyestrain*: Eyestrain is the most frequently mentioned problem caused by lighting, or the lack thereof. It can be caused by one or several of the following conditions: inadequate illumination; glare; flicker; uncorrected refractive errors (need for eyeglasses); and a non-ergonomic positioning of the visual task.

   Eyestrain can lead to headaches and fatigue, which in turn add to stress. Let's examine glare first. Glare can be diffuse, specula, or direct. Veiling reflections off a magazine page can cause discomfort, or even disability (the inability to perform a task; in this case, reading the printed text). Glare is never desirable, and a lot of work has gone into determining how to reduce it, especially in offices with VDTs. Unfortunately, through ignorance or over-zealousness, many offices are now too dark for general task work (a trait shared by many residences). Research has shown that limiting ceiling luminance ratios to below 5:1 helps a lot

2. *Flicker*: Flicker is well known for causing eyestrain. Humans can perceive flicker at frequencies as high as 200 Hz, based on measured physiologic responses in the retina. Flicker is most apparent in the peripheral areas of vision, where the rods are concentrated; however, if the frequency is low enough, the cones have sufficient time to react, and then flicker really becomes objectionable because it is cognitively noticeable as a distraction. Gas-discharge lamps such as fluorescents and metal-halides usually flicker at 120 Hz (twice the power line frequency) because their arcs are extinguished at every zero-crossing of current. The newer electronic ballasts can drive these lamps at 25 - 40

KHz, well beyond visual and audible perception by humans (but perhaps not so for certain pets). Incandescent lamps also flicker sinusoid ally at 120 Hz, but the filament remains hot enough for it not to be noticeable by most people. However, there are some halogen lamps with integral diodes which exhibit severe flicker; they can also audibly hum or click.

3. *Noise*: As mentioned above, flicker and noise often accompany each other. Here the lighting system is to blame, not the light itself. All lamp ballasts and transformers produce some noise at harmonics of the line frequency. Noise produces stress in humans. Currently, of all the types of ballasts and transformers for all the different lamp technologies, only some fluorescent ballasts are "rated" for noise; there is no certification requirement -- a scandalous situation.
4. *Fears*: This section discusses issues of some controversy, some of which are being aggressively researched for health risks. Non- technical readers are strongly advised to acquire a basic understanding of risk assessment, and are directed to an excellent place to start.

UV and Skin Cancer Risk from Lighting

There have been many claims for and against skin exposure to UV. The CIE defines three bands of UV, listed in order of increasing energy:

- UV-A 380nm - 315nm
- UV-B 315nm - 280nm
- UV-C 280nm - 100nm

UV-C will quickly kill most micro-organisms, and is used for that purpose. Human skin uses UV-B to produce vitamin D3, which is needed for maintenance of proper calcium: phosphorus balance. Most milk is fortified with vitamin D3, which seems to have obviated the need for skin exposure (assuming person drinks fortified milk). UV-B is strongly suspected as the cause of lens yellowing and cataract formation, besides carcinoma and melanoma. Benefits and hazards of UV-A have not been thoroughly researched. UV exposure can have systemic effects on the immune system. On the other hand, there may still be a minimum daily requirement for UV exposure. There is evidence that certain wavelengths of UV-A and blue light can repair damage to DNA caused by UV-B also, the greater transparency to UV of the eyes of children may play a role in their physical development.

Quality of Lighting

As we developed lighting and other building technologies, we gained control of our immediate environment, but in many cases, we also became isolated from the natural environment. There are some major differences between the outdoors lit environment and the typical office lighting. First, the outdoors is more brightly lit -- much more. The luminance from the sky alone (sun blocked) can exceed 10,000lux; with direct sunlight added, luminance can exceed 100,000 lux. Compare this to a "brightly lit" office at 1000lux (93 foot-candles). Second, the light from the sky is very uniform and very diffuse; it is almost like being inside a giant fluorescent tube. Third, the amount of light varies smoothly over the course of the day. Fourth, the sky is blue (colour temp > 6000K); not many offices have blue walls and ceilings (for good reasons...). Fifth, the colour temperature changes smoothly throughout the course of the day, rarely dropping below 5000K (at noon), then increasing to over 10,000K at dusk. Lastly, there is significantly more UV present, at all wavelengths.

Recommendations

A. ***General Recommendations:*** Indoor lighting should not fall below 500 lux as an absolute minimum; 1000 lux is better. Day lighting should be used as much as possible, both for its superior quality, and its energy-saving potential. Good day lighting is difficult to implement, however; light shelves are becoming an increasingly popular architectural approach. High (>9ft) ceilings also help a lot. Use lamps with a colour temperature of 5000 - 6000 K, full- spectrum optional. If there is concern about UV exposure, buy filters. Eyeglass wearers (especially the elderly) should have untimed lenses with anti-reflective (AR) coatings.

B. ***Lighting for the Vision Impaired and Elderly:*** Use enough illumination. Persons with macular degeneration perform much better with illumination exceeding 5000 lux.Make all lighting transitions from one space to another as gradually as possible; the elderly take longer to adapt. If someone moves from a brightly-lit space into a darker corridor, he or she will not adapt in time, but will be effectively blinded. This might be why so many falls occur in hallways and stairwells. Taking extra care to avoid sources of glare will help to reduce the disability glare caused by intra-ocular scattering. In a few cases, people with very cloudy eye conditions can improve their visual clarity and contrast sensitivity by wearing "blue-blocking" lenses or filters

C. ***Night Shift Lighting*:** Campaign against rotating shifts, and avoid the night shift. Give night-shift workers as much light as possible, preferably above 2500lux, while being careful not to cause glare. Promote the use of sleep-phase shifting, so workers can be in sync with their environment.

7.1.7 Adverse Health Effects of Thermal Radiation

There are various health effects seen on human body due to the thermal radiation which are as follows:

- It causes skin damage. It burns/heats surface of the skin and tissues immediately below.
- It is very dangerous to the eye (because retina is very sensitive to it). It can cause temporary blindness if it is intense or can cause permanent eye damage if it is very intense.
- Redness and burns to the skin. Retina burns and development of eye cataracts over time.
- It causes pain and inflammation to the surface of the eye leading to temporary blindness.
- There is high risk of skin cancer due to radiation.
- Continuous expose to thermal radiation causes internal organ damage and can be fatal.
- Also thermal radiation causes loss of weight, appetite bleeding and discoloured spots on skin.
- Thermal radiation causes dead layer of cells on the surface of skin.
- Other thermal radiation effects includes :
  1. Hair loss.
  2. Blistering and ulceration of skin.
  3. Nausea, vomiting and diarrhoea

4. Dermatitis
5. Anaemia due red blood cell damage
6. Infertility

7.1.8 Adverse Health Effects of Ionizing and Non-Ionizing Radiation

A. Adverse health effects of ionizing radiation: Various sources of ionizing radiation causes different health effects as per the source:

1. ***Alpha particles:*** This alpha particles causes to form dead layer of cells on the surface of skin.
2. ***Beta particles:*** This particles penetrates through skin and causes to damage to living tissues.
3. ***X-rays, Gamma rays and Neutrons:*** This type of electromagnetic radiation causes following acute effects-
   (a) Hair loss.
   (b) Blistering and ulceration of skin.
   (c) Nausea, vomiting and diarrhoea
   (d) Dermatitis
   (e) Anaemia due red blood cell damage
   (f) Infertility
   (g) Cataracts
   (h) Reduced immune system due to white blood cell damage
4. ***Chronic effects due to ionizing radiation***
   (a) Cancer
   (b) Genetic mutations
   (c) Birth defects

B. Adverse health effects of non-ionizing radiation: Various sources of ionizing radiation causes different health effects as per the source:

1. ***Ultra-violet (UV):*** This causes
   (a) Redness and burns to the skin
   (b) Pain and inflammation to the surface of eye leading to temporary blindness known as photo keratitis.

(c) Increases risk of skin cancer

(d) Premature aging of the skin

2. ***Visible light:*** This is particularly dangerous to eyes because retina is very sensitive to it. It can cause temporary blindness or permanent eye damage.

3. ***Infra-red (IR):*** IR health effects include redness and burns to the skin, retinal burns and development of eye cataracts overtime.

4. ***Microwaves:*** Microwaves are absorbed and cause internal heating of the skin. High dose cause internal organ damage and can be fatal.

5. ***Radio waves:*** Radio waves absorbed by body and cause internal heating of body and instant skin burns and eye damage.

7.2 Permissible Threshold Exposure Limit

Whenever you work with a chemical you need to understand the hazards posed by the chemical in order to perform a proper risk assessment. You might discover that the material is flammable, or explosive, or may react with common substances such as water, air, or bleach. Another piece of information that you may run across is the exposure limits for the chemical. These limits provide very useful information on the health risks associated with the chemical. But you need to understand what the numbers are saying, and know their limitations. Before describing the main occupational exposure values, here are some key points to consider:

- Occupational exposure limits have been set by numerous organizations, but values tend to be reported only for the most common industrial chemicals and these are mainly based on inhalation hazards. The lack of a published exposure limit should not be interpreted as meaning that hazards do not exist.
- Laboratories differ significantly from industrial settings where exposures are often continuous throughout the work period. In labs there is the potential for exposure to a large

number of chemicals but exposures, if they do occur, tend to be of short duration.

- Exposure limits, with the exceptions of the legally enforceable PELs (see below), are guidelines and are useful when taking a risk-based approach, but it is prudent to avoid – through proper use of engineering controls, personal protective equipment, and administrative controls – any unnecessary exposure.
- You may find different exposure limits for the same chemicals. Each organization has its own method for developing the exposure values so some will be more conservative than others.

Permissible Exposure Limits (PELs)

The Occupational Health and Safety Administration (OSHA) has set permissible exposure limits (PELs) on the amount or concentration of a substance in the air. The limits may also contain a skin designation that serves as a warning of potential cutaneous absorption that should be prevented in order to avoid exceeding the absorbed dose received by inhalation at the permissible exposure level (PEL). These limits are enforceable by law. Most OSHA PELs are based on an 8-hour work shift of a 40-hour workweek time-weighted average (TWA) exposure that an employee may be exposed to for a working lifetime without adverse effects. In most laboratory settings exposures are of short duration so time-weighted averages are difficult to exceed. Some of the PELs are listed as ceiling values – concentrations above which a worker should never be exposed, or short-term exposure limits (STELs) –average concentrations which should not be exceeded over a 15 minute time period. It is important to note that the PELs tend to be higher than other published values.

Threshold Limit Value (TLV)

Threshold Limit Values (TLV) are occupational exposure limits set by the American Conference of Governmental Industrial Hygienists (ACGIH). The Time-Weighted Average TLV (TLV-TWA) is an airborne concentration of a gas or particle to which most workers can be exposed on a daily basis for a working lifetime without adverse effect (assuming an average exposure on the basis of a 8h/day, 40h/week work schedule).

Physical hazard exposure limit

Temperature

Table 7.1 ACGIH Screening Criteria for Heat Stress Exposure (WBGT values in °C) for 8 hour work day five days per week with conventional breaks

Allocation of Work in a Work/Rest Cycle	TLV®				Action Limit			
	Light	Moderate	Heavy	Very Heavy	Light	Moderate	Heavy	Very Heavy
75-100%	31.0	28.0	--	--	28.0	25.0	--	--
50-75%	31.0	29.0	27.5	--	28.5	26.0	24.0	--
25-50%	32.0	30.0	29.0	28.0	29.5	27.0	25.5	24.5
0-25%	32.5	31.5	30.5	30.0	30.0	29.0	28.0	27.0

Notes: Table is intended as a screening tool to evaluate if a heat stress situation may exist.
Assumes 8-hour workdays in a 5-day workweek with conventional breaks.
TLVs assume that workers exposed to these conditions are adequately hydrated, are not taking medication, are wearing lightweight clothing, and are in generally good health.
Examples of work loads
Rest - sitting (quietly or with moderate arm movements)
Light work - sitting or standing to control machines; performing light hand or arm work (e.g. using a table saw); occasional walking; driving
Moderate work - walking about with moderate lifting and pushing or pulling; walking at moderate pace; e.g. scrubbing in a standing position
Heavy work - pick and shovel work, digging, carrying, pushing/pulling heavy loads; walking at fast pace; e.g. carpenter sawing by hand
Very Heavy - very intense activity at fast to maximum pace; e.g. shovelling wet sand

Table 7.2 Humidor and Thermal Comfort

Humidor Range(°C)	Degrees of Comfort
20 - 29	Comfortable
30 - 39	Varying degrees of discomfort
40 - 45	Uncomfortable
46 and Over	Many types of labour must be restricted

Lighting

Examples of industrial and office tasks and the recommended light levels are in the table below.

Table 7.3 Recommended Illumination Levels

Type of Activity	Ranges of Illuminations (Lux)**
Public spaces with dark surroundings	20-50
Simple orientation for short temporary visits	50-100
Working spaces where visual tasks are only occasionally performed	100-200
Performance of visual tasks of high contrast or large scale	200-500
Performance of visual tasks of medium contrast or small size	500-1000
Performance of visual tasks of low contrast or very small size	1000-2000
Performance of visual tasks of low contrast and very small size over a prolonged period	2000-5000
Performance of very prolonged and exacting visual tasks	5000-10000

Noise

Table 7.4 Hearing Disability Calculation using the American Medical Association Formula

Frequency, Hz	Hearing Threshold Level, dB	
	Left Ear	Right Ear
500	30	15
1000	45	25
2000	60	45
3000	85	55
Sum	220	140
Average	55	35
Low fence	25	25
Exceeds low fence	30	10
%Impairment	45	15
Disability	[45 + (5x15)]/6 = 20%	

Vibration

Table Maximum satisfactory magnitudes of vibration with respect to human response

Place	Time	Satisfactory Magnitude pp. (mm/s)
Residential	Day (08.00 – 18.00, Mon-Fri & 08.00 – 13.00, Sat) Night (23.00 - 07.00) Other (times not included above)	6.0 to 10.00 2.0 4.5
Offices	Any time	14.0
Workshops	Any time	14.0

Ultraviolet and ionizing radiation

One Sievert is a large dose. The recommended TLV is average annual dose of 0.05 vs. (50 Ms).

The effects of being exposed to large doses of radiation at one time (acute exposure) vary with the dose. Here are some examples:

10 Vs. - Risk of death within days or weeks

1 Vs. - Risk of cancer later in life (5 in 100)

100 Ms - Risk of cancer later in life (5 in 1000)

50 Ms - TLV for annual dose for radiation workers in any one year

20 Ms - TLV for annual average dose, averaged over five years

The Threshold Limit Values (TLVs) published by the ACGIH (American Conference of Governmental Industrial Hygienists) are used in many jurisdictions occupational exposure limits or guidelines:

20 Ms - TLV for average annual dose for radiation workers, averaged over five years

1 Ms - Recommended annual dose limit for general public (ICRP - International Commission on Radiological Protection).

Chemical hazard

Chemical Name	Potential Health Effects/Symptoms Associated with Toxicity (Note: not a complete listing of symptoms
Methylene chloride	• Mild central nervous system depressant. May cause headache, nausea, dizziness, drowsiness, incoordination and confusion, unconsciousness and death. • Causes skin and eye irritation.
Isopropyl alcohol (2-propanol)	• Mild central nervous system depressant. High vapour concentrations may cause headache, nausea, dizziness, drowsiness, incoordination, and confusion. Very high exposures may result in unconsciousness and death.

Contd...

Chemical Name	Potential Health Effects/Symptoms Associated with Toxicity (Note: not a complete listing of symptoms
	• May be irritating to the respiratory tract. • Causes eye irritation. • Swallowing or vomiting of the liquid may cause aspiration (breathing) into the lungs.
Acetone	• Mild central nervous system depressant. • Very high concentrations may cause headache, nausea, dizziness, drowsiness, incoordination and confusion. • Causes eye irritation. • Swallowing or vomiting of the liquid may result in aspiration into the lungs.
l-Limonene	• Causes moderate skin irritation. • May cause allergic skin reaction.
Acetaldehyde	• The vapour is irritating to the respiratory tract. May cause lung injury. These effects may be delayed. • Causes severe eye irritation.
Hydrogen peroxide (>35%)	• May be fatal if swallowed.

Assessment of Long-Term Exposures to Toxic Substances in Air

Because airborne exposure varies greatly over time and between individual workers, occupational hygienists should adopt sampling strategies which recognize the inherent statistical nature of assessing exposure. This analysis indicates that the traditional practice of testing 'compliance' with occupational exposure limits (OELs) should be discarded. Rather, it is argued that acceptable exposure should be defined with reference to the exposure distribution. Regarding the many statistical issues which come into play, it is concluded that hygienists should continue to apply the log-normal model for summarizing and testing data. However, sampling designs should move away from methods which are biased (e.g., sampling only the worst case) and which rely upon job title and observation as the primary means of assigning workers into groups. Since exposure data often lack independence (e.g., owing to the autocorrelation of serial measurements) and there exist large differences in exposure between workers in the same job group, random sampling designs should be adopted. It is also shown that the relationship between the mean of a log-normal distribution and exposures in the right tail allows one to evaluate simultaneously the mean exposure and the maximum frequency with which exposures exceed the OEL.

Investigation of the biological concepts relies heavily upon a conceptual model which depicts the exposure-response continuum as a sequence of time series related to exposure, burden, damage and risk. Analysis of the linkages between these processes identifies two kinetic conditions which are necessary if variability of exposure is to affect appreciably the individual's risk of chronic disease. First, the variation of exposure from interval to interval must be efficiently translated into burden and damage (no damping), and second, during periods of intense exposure the relationship between burden and damage must be non-linear (curving upwards). On the basis of current knowledge it appears that relatively few chronic toxicants satisfy both these conditions. Even for those substances which cause damage only when a threshold is exceeded, a statistical argument suggests that the maximum risk can still be related to the mean exposure received over time.

It is concluded that the risk of chronic disease generally depends upon the mean exposure received by the individual worker over time. Thus, the sampling strategy must allow the distribution of individual mean exposures to be characterized across the population at risk. It follows from this paradigm for assessing exposures that relatively little effort should be devoted to the evaluation of short-term 'peak' exposures since such transients are unlikely to exert undue influence on long-term effects. Regarding short-term effects it is argued that evaluation of exposures to acutely toxic agents should rely upon assessment and control of the source rather than of exposure per se.

Finally, three approaches are evaluated for testing exposures relative to limits: the test of compliance; a test of the frequency of excursions; and a test of the mean exposure: By several objective criteria it is shown that the traditional test of compliance offers a poor tool for prospective assessment. While both of the other approaches allow rigorous testing to be conducted, evaluation of the mean1 exposure appears superior on the grounds of statistical power and the relationship between outcome and the long-term hazard. However, investigation of the underlying bases for OELs indicates that exposure limits can allow more risk to prevail than is generally presumed and the variation of exposure among workers in a group can be large. Thus, it may be necessary to incorporate safety factors into OELs prior to testing mean exposures.

7.3 Long Term and Short Term Effects of Exposure

Assessing Exposures

Lead-related Construction Tasks and Their Presumed 8-hour TWA Exposure Levels

> 50 to 500 µg/m3

Manual demolition

Dry manual scraping

Dry manual sanding

Heat gun use

Power tool cleaning with dust collection systems

Spray painting with lead paint

> 500 µg/m3 to 2,500 µg/m3

Using lead-containing mortar

Lead burning

Rivet busting

Power tool cleaning without dust collection systems

Cleanup of dry expendable abrasive blasting jobs

Abrasive blasting enclosure movement and removal

> 2,500 µg/m3

Abrasive blasting

Welding

Torch cutting

Torch burning

7.4 Preventive and Control Measures

Lead is a cumulative and persistent toxic substance. Lead-related health effects may result from low levels of exposure over prolonged periods of time. Engineering controls and good work practices must be used where feasible to minimize employee exposure to lead. At a minimum, exposures must not exceed the OSHA interim final PEL of 50 micrograms per cubic meter of air (50 mg/m3) averaged over an 8-hour period. When feasible engineering controls and work practice controls cannot reduce worker exposure to lead at or below 50 mg/m3, respirators must be used to supplement engineering and work practice controls. A competent person should review all site operations and stipulate the specific engineering controls and work practices designed to reduce worker exposure to lead. Engineering measures include local and general exhaust ventilation, process and equipment modification, material substitution, component replacement, and isolation or automation. Examples of recommended engineering controls that can be used to reduce worker exposure to lead are as follows: Exhaust Ventilation Power tools used for the removal of lead-based paint should be equipped with dust collection shrouds or other attachments exhausted through a high-efficiency particulate air (HEPA) vacuum system. Operations such as welding, cutting/burning or heating should be provided with local exhaust ventilation. HEPA vacuums should be used during cleanup activities.

For abrasive blasting operations where full containment exists or is required, the containment structure should be designed to optimize the flow of ventilation air past the workers, so that the airborne concentration of lead is reduced and the visibility is increased. The affected area should be maintained under negative pressure to reduce the chances that lead dust will contaminate areas outside the enclosure. A containment structure should be equipped with dust collection and an air cleaning device to control emissions of particulate matter to the environment. Enclosure/Encapsulation Lead-based paint can be made inaccessible either by encapsulating it with a material that bonds to the surface, such as acrylic or epoxy coating or flexible wall coverings, or by enclosing it using systems such as gypsum wallboard, plywood panelling, and aluminium, vinyl or wood exterior siding. Floors coated with lead-based paint can be covered using vinyl tile or linoleum flooring. The building owner or other responsible person should oversee the custodial and maintenance staffs and contractors with regard to all activities that involve enclosed or encapsulated lead-based paint. This will minimize potential inadvertent release of lead during maintenance, renovation or demolition. Substitution Zinc-containing primers covered by an epoxy intermediate coat and polyurethane topcoat are commonly used instead of lead-containing coatings. Mobile hydraulic shears can be substituted for torch cutting under certain circumstances. Surface preparation equipment, such as needle guns with multiple reciprocating needles completely enclosed within an adjustable shroud, can be substituted for abrasive blasting under certain operations. The shroud captures dust and debris at the cutting edge and can be equipped with a HEPA vacuum filtration system with a self-drumming feature. One such commercial unit can remove lead-based paint from flat steel and concrete surfaces, outside edges, inside corners, and pipes. One who is capable of identifying existing and predictable lead hazards in the surroundings or working conditions and who has authorization to take prompt corrective measures to eliminate them? Chemical strippers used primarily on the exterior of buildings, surfaces involving carvings or melding, or intricate iron works—can be used in place of hand scraping using a heat gun. Chemical removal generates less airborne lead dust; however, these strippers can be hazardous.

The safety data sheets (SDSs) for the products used must be reviewed by the employer for information on worker exposure hazards from the chemical ingredients and protective measures recommended by the manufacturer. Component Replacement Lead-base painted building components (e.g., windows, doors and trim) can be replaced either with new components free of lead-containing paint or with the same components after the paint has been removed off-site. Replacement is a permanent solution. Process/Equipment Modification Brush/roller application of lead paints or other lead-containing coatings is a safer method than spraying. This method of application introduces little or no paint mist into the air where the mist can present a lead inhalation hazard. (Note: There is a ban on the use of lead-based paint in residential housing.) Non-silica containing abrasive (e.g., steel or iron shot/grit) should be used, where practical, instead of sand in abrasive blasting operations. When sand is used, the free silica portion of the dust presents a significant respiratory health hazard. Blasting techniques that are less dusty than abrasive blasting and that can be effective under some conditions include (1) hydro- or wet-blasting (using high-pressure water with or without abrasive, or surrounding the blast nozzle with a ring of water) and (2) vacuum blasting where a vacuum hood for material removal is positioned around the exterior of the blasting nozzle. Heat guns used to remove lead-based paints in residential housing units should be of the flameless electrical softener type. Heat guns should have electronically controlled temperature settings to allow usage below 700 degrees F. Heat guns should be equipped with various nozzles to cover all common applications and to limit the heated work area. When using abrasive blasting with vacuum hood on exterior building surfaces, care should be taken that the configuration of the heads on the blasting nozzle match the configuration of the substrate, so that the vacuum is effective in containing debris.

Since HEPA vacuum cleaners can be used to clean surfaces other than just floors, operators should have attachments appropriate for use on unusual surfaces. The proper use of brushes of various sizes and crevice and angular tools, when needed, will enhance the quality of the HEPA-vacuuming process and help reduce the amount of lead dust released into the air. Isolation although it is not feasible to completely enclose and ventilate some abrasive blasting operations, it is possible to isolate many operations to help reduce the potential for exposure to lead. Isolation, in this instance, consists of keeping employees not involved in the blasting operations as far away as possible from the work area. By placing the employees a greater distance from the source of lead exposure, their exposures will be reduced.

7.5 Pre-Employment and Periodic Medical Examination of Workers

Workers medical assessment specifies as pre and periodic medical examinations. It is one of the most important aspect in placing the workers for suitable jobs. Further it is essential to assess the worker health status periodically to justify that the worker is in good health to perform the work effectively. Biological monitoring ensures the workers physical fitness to perform the job productively and efficiently which intern reduces the health expenditure, absenteeism and turn over in industries.

The medical testing will be very specifically focused to assess the health status based on the exposures. The worker will be given a report based on the reports and the company will be given a special report based on the worker health assessment reports and hazard identification.

There are two main purposes of pre-employment medical examinations:

1. **To provide base-line health data:** This is important for assessment of the effectiveness of preventive measures at work. For example, where the hearing threshold of a worker, which is normal before employment in a noisy occupation, is found to have increased after employment, this possibly indicates noise-induced hearing loss and a review of the hearing protection measures would be required. On the other hand, if the pre-employment hearing threshold of the ascertain whether the worker's high hearing threshold after employment is due to excessive noise exposure at work or to his own hearing problem before employment. Pre-employment health data is also important in substantiating or negating employees' compensation claims since it provides evidence of the health status of claimants before employment.
2. **To ensure Medical fitness for work:** Pre-employment medical examination identify those person who are medically unfit for employment in particular occupations. Persons with certain underlying medical conditions are particularly vulnerable to the effects of certain health hazards and are not suitable for employment in work with such exposures.

   Workers may fail to meet the specific health requirements for particular jobs, so they have to take the safely without risk to others.

   Periodic medical examinations aim to detect susceptible workers for whom corrective actions are required before they develop overt occupational diseases. For example, a lead worker with a high blood lead level should be suspended from work temporarily to stop further exposure to lead and to receive necessary medical treatment. Meanwhile, safety and health measures at work should be reviewed for necessary remedial actions. The frequency of periodic medical examinations depends on the nature of the occupational hazards. For most hazardous exposures, however, these examinations are conducted annually.

Type of services to be conducted periodically

1. **Audiometry test**
   - (i) If the noise levels are drawn are very high in the respective areas in the industry or construction site.
   - (ii) Audio graph will be drawn and provided individually.
   - (iii) Target the workers who are exposed to noise.
   - (iv) Check regular assessment
2. **Blood Analysis**
   - (i) Full blood count
   - (ii) Liver functioning well
   - (iii) Blood test report
   - (iv) Remedies and suggestions are to be given.
   - (v) Fasting blood sugar levels will be checked
3. **Fitness to work assessment**
   - (i) Factory visit will be done as a preliminary step to identify the hazards in the specific.
   - (ii) Factory visit.
4. **Medical examination and provision report**
   - (i) Based on the factory visit findings the workers will be physically examined by a qualified occupational physician at the company premises.
   - (ii) The workers will be selected based on the identified occupational hazards.
   - (iii) They will be subjected to blood testing, audiometric examination, lung function testing or vision testing by competent staff.
5. **Physical examination**
   - (i) This includes a physical examination
   - (ii) Blood pressure.
   - (iii) BMI checking

6. Lungs functioning testing

(i) If the working premises are dusty or if the workers are exposed to chemicals.

(ii) FVC/FEC/ PEFR reports will be obtained

(iii) Target workers who are working & exposed to dust.

7. Vision testing

Based on the visual acuity, the workers will be referred to an optician and if required free spectacles will be provided.

Medical Examination requirement

The requirements of medical examinations depend on the nature of the hazardous exposures of workers. In general, the doctor will take a detailed occupational and medical history, conduct a physical examination and prescribe a range of ancillary laboratory and/or radiological investigations such as urine test, blood test, X-ray, lung function test and audiometric test.

Benefits to the industry

(i) Will be able to legally valid document /individually and company based

(ii) Will be able to reduce the health budget in the industry as it contains the noise induced hearing losses mitigating recommendations.

(iii) Compliance to the National safety & Health law.

(iv) Added value in ISO /OSHA certifications.

(v) Increase profitability by reducing absenteeism, occupational accidents and occupational diseases.

7.6 Medical Surveillance and Health Records

Medical Surveillance

Objective

The primary purpose of the medical surveillance program is to identify medical conditions that could lead to an occupational disease. The secondary objective is to assure compliance with federal and state regulations which require medical monitoring when employees use certain materials.

Purpose

The purpose of medical surveillance is for the early identification of conditions, if any, that could present an increased risk of adverse health effects related to the task being performed.

Based on the type of work being performed, including consideration of factors such as the duration of the task, the materials being used, and the potential for exposure, medical surveillance is either recommended or required for the job.

Specific test results and other personal medical information generated by these exams will be kept confidential between the employee and the physician. The physician will determine the scope of the exam, then inform the supervisor of their recommendations based on the exam results. The supervisor will discuss these recommendations, if any, with the employee. The employee can contact the physician who performs the exam with any questions regarding the test results.

According to federal law, employees have the right to request copies of their medical or exposure records at any time by contacting their supervisor or Human Resources.

Scope

This section pertains to medical surveillance of employees and students related to the use of chemicals, physical agents (noise, radiation), or animal contact. Medical surveillance, as described in this section, does not include discussion of fitness for duty exams (e.g. Campus Police Officer, Emergency Responder, etc.)

General principles

Medical surveillance includes, where appropriate, pre-assignment and periodical medical examinations. It also includes, where appropriate, medical examinations upon resumption of work after a prolonged absence for health reasons, and upon and after termination of work involving exposure to chemicals.

Medical surveillance, conducted by an approved medical practitioner, should be used as part of overall health surveillance, in accordance with the objectives and principles of the Occupational Health Services Recommendation, 1985 (No.

171). Health surveillance should also include, where appropriate, simple techniques for the early detection of effects on health. These could include examination and questioning about health complaints.

Where necessary, the employer, or the institution competent under national law and practice, should arrange, through a method which accords with national law and practice, medical surveillance of workers:

(a) For the assessment of the health of workers in relation to risks caused by exposure to chemicals.

(b) For the early diagnosis of work-related diseases and injuries caused by exposure to hazardous chemicals.

(c) For the assessment of the workers' ability to wear or use required respiratory or other personal protective equipment.

In the case of exposure of workers to specific hazards, medical and health surveillance should include, where appropriate, any examination and investigations which may be necessary to detect exposure levels and early biological effects and responses.

Medical surveillance is necessary where

(a) It is required by national law whenever workers are liable to be exposed to chemicals hazardous to health.

(b) The employer is advised by an occupational health service that it is necessary as part of the protection of workers exposed to chemicals hazardous to health, given special attention to pregnant and breastfeeding women and other susceptible workers.

(c) Atmospheric or biological monitoring show that there could be effects on the health of a worker because of exposure to chemicals at work and medical surveillance will assist early detection of ill effects.

Exposure to the following types of chemicals may be appropriate for medical surveillance

(a) Chemicals that have a recognised systemic toxicity, i.e. an insidious poisonous effect;

(b) Chemicals known to cause chronic effects, e.g. occupational asthma;

(c) Chemicals known to cause severe dermatitis;

(d) Chemicals that are known or suspected carcinogens;

Health Records

A health record must be kept for all employees under health surveillance.

Records are important because they allow links to be made between exposure and any health effects. Health records, or a copy, should be kept in a suitable form for at least 40 years from the date of last entry because often there is a long period between exposure and onset of ill health

What information should be included in health record?

Individual, up-to-date health records must be kept for each employee placed under health surveillance. These should include details about the employee and the health surveillance procedures relating to them.

Employee details should include

- Surname
- Forename(s)
- Gender
- Date of birth
- Permanent address, including post code
- National Insurance number
- Date present employment started

Recorded details of each health surveillance check should include

- The date they were carried out and by whom
- The outcome of the test/check
- The decision made by the occupational health professional in terms of fitness for task and any restrictions required. This should be factual and only relate to the employee's functional ability and fitness for specific work, with any advised restrictions.

The record should be kept in a format that it can be linked with other information (e.g., with any workplace exposure measurements).

If you are collecting an historical record of jobs or tasks completed during current employment, involving exposure to identified substances requiring health surveillance it is useful to store them with this record.

For some exposures, all you need to do is set up and maintain records that may be viewed alongside other information, such as air sampling or biological monitoring results. This is the case, eg. With work involving:

- Rubber manufacturing and processing, giving rise to rubber process dust and rubber fume - except health surveillance/medical surveillance needed for rubber manufacturing.
- Leather dust in boot and shoe manufacture

It is good practice to offer individual employees a copy of their health record when they leave your employment. If your company changes hands, consider offering the health record to the individual employee, and/or to the new occupational health service provider. Make sure that health records are stored securely.

What health Record should contain

Health records are different to medical records in that they should not contain confidential medical information. Health records and medical records must therefore be kept separate to avoid any breaches of medical confidentiality.

Any personal medical information should be kept in confidence and held by the occupational health professional responsible for the health surveillance programme.

Medical records are compiled by a doctor or nurse and may contain information obtained from the individual during the course of health surveillance. This information may include clinical notes, biological results and other information related to health issues not associated with work. This information is confidential and should not be disclosed without the consent of the individual.

The occupational health (OH) professional may obtain data as the result of an immunisation programme (for example, blood titres or 'non responder' information). This information will be provided to the employee and should not be given to the employer. It will be kept in confidence by the OH professional and should only made known to the employer with the employee's consent.

The doctor or nurse should only provide employers with information on fitness to work and any restrictions that may apply in that respect. Employees can have access to their own medical record through a written request under the data protection act. These details can only be released to third parties, such as the employer, on receipt of the informed written consent of the employee, or by a court order.

CHAPTER 8

Fundamentals of First Aid

8.1 Introduction to First Aid

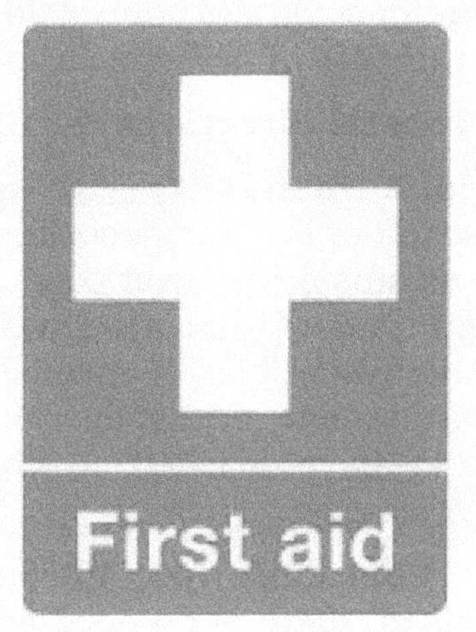

First aid is the immediate care given to a person who has been injured or suddenly taken ill. It includes self-help and home care if medical assistance is not available or is delayed. It also includes well-selected words of encouragement, evidence of willingness to help, and promotion of confidence by demonstration of competence.

The person giving first aid, the first-alder, deals with the whole situation, the injured person, and the injury or illness. He knows what not to do as well as what to do; he avoids errors that are frequently made by untrained persons through well-meant but misguided efforts. He knows, too, that his first aid knowledge and skill can mean the difference between life and death, between temporary and permanent disability, and between rapid recovery and long hospitalization.

A. Need for first aid training

Statistics show that accidents are the leading cause of death among persons from 1 year old to 38 years old; thereafter, accidents are one of the leading causes. The annual cost of medical attention, the loss of earning ability due to temporary or permanent impairment, the direct property damage, and the insurance costs amount to many billions of dollars each year, not to mention the toll in pain, suffering, disability, and personal tragedy.

Added to the grim accident statistics is the fact that the pattern of medical care has changed. Individuals today require, and should demand, the best possible care. Equipment for diagnosis and treatment, which is needed to provide such care, is usually at a hospital. Moreover, the growing population and expanding health needs have not been balanced by a proportional increase in numbers of doctors, nurses, and allied health workers. It is not enough to say, "Call the doctor"; a doctor may not be available to come to the scene of the emergency.

Value of first aid training

First aid training is of value in both preventing and treating sudden illness or accidental injury and in caring for large numbers of persons caught in a natural disaster.

General directions for first aid

As a first-aider, you may encounter a variety of problem situations. Your decisions and actions will vary according to the circumstances that produced the accident or sudden illness, the number of persons involved, the immediate environment, and the availability of medical assistance, emergency dressings and equipment, and help from others. You will need to adapt what you have learned to the situation at hand or will need to improvise.

Sometimes, prompt action is needed to save a life. At other times, there is no need for haste. Efforts in the latter case will be directed toward preventing further injury, obtaining assistance, and reassuring the victim, who may be emotionally upset and apprehensive, as well as in pain.

First aid begins with action, which in itself has a calming effect. If there are multiple injuries or if several persons are hurt, priorities must be set. If you are the first-aider in charge you should enlist the help of bystanders to make telephone calls, to direct traffic, to keep others at a distance if necessary, to position safety flares in case of highway accidents, and so on. You should provide life support to victims with life-threatening injuries, attending first to those suffering from stoppage of breathing and then to those with severe hemorrhaging. You can then turn to those with less critical injuries.

Telephone or have someone else telephone the appropriate authorities regarding the accident. The police department or the high-way patrol is a good first contact, but the circumstances surrounding the accident should be a guide as to whom to call. You should always have a list of emergency telephone numbers available. If the numbers are not readily available, ask the operator for assistance. Describe the problem, indicate what is being done, and ask for whatever help you think is needed, such as an ambulance, the fire department, the rescue squad, or utility company personnel. Give your name, the location of the accident, the number of persons involved, and the telephone number where you can be reached. Do not hang up the receiver until after the other party hangs up, because he may wish to clarify some information.

8.2 Burns

1 What causes burns?

You can get burned by heat, fire, radiation, sunlight, electricity, chemicals or hot or boiling water. There are 3 degrees of burns:

First-degree burns are red and painful. They swell a little. They turn white when you press on the skin. The skin over the burn may peel off after 1 or 2 days.

Second-degree burns are thicker burns, are very painful and typically produce blisters on the skin. The skin is very red or splotchy, and may be very swollen.

Third-degree burns cause damage to all layers of the skin. The burned skin looks white or charred. These burns may cause little or no pain because the nerves and tissue in the skin are damaged.

How long does it take for burns to heal?

First-degree burns usually heal in 3 to 6 days.

Second-degree burns usually heal in 2 to 3 weeks.

Third-degree burns usually take a very long time to heal.

How are burns treated?

The treatment depends on what kind of burn you have.

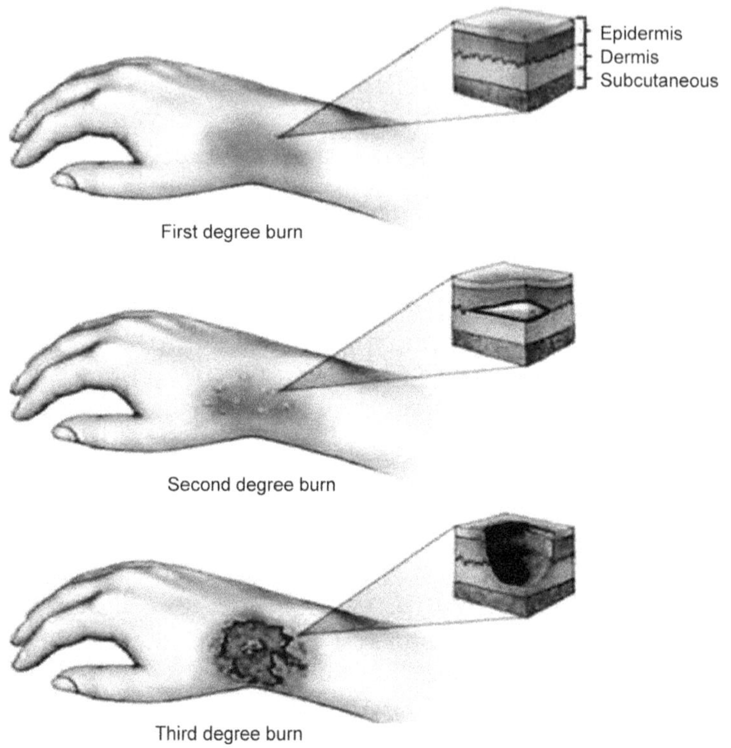

See a doctor if

A first- or second-degree burn covers an area larger than 2 to 3 inches in diameter. The burn is on your face, over a major joint (such as the knee or shoulder), on the hands, feet or genitals.

The burn is a third-degree burn, which requires immediate medical attention.

First-degree burn

Soak the burn in cool water for at least 5 minutes. The cool water helps reduce swelling by pulling heat away from the burned skin. Treat the burn with a skin care product that protects and heals skin, such as aloe Vera cream or an antibiotic ointment. You can wrap a dry gauze bandage loosely around the burn. This will protect the area and keep the air off of it.

Take an over-the-counter pain reliever, such as acetaminophen (one brand name: Tylenol), ibuprofen (some brand names: Advil, Motrin) or naproxen (brand name: Aleve), to help with the pain. Ibuprofen and naproxen will also help with swelling.

Second-degree burn

Soak the burn in cool water for 15 minutes. If the burned area is small, put cool, clean, wet clothes on the burn for a few minutes every day. Then put on an antibiotic cream, or other creams or ointments prescribed by your doctor. Cover the burn with a dry non-stick dressing (for example, Telfair) held in place with gauze or tape. Checks with your doctor's office to make sure you are up-to-date on tetanus shots.

Change the dressing every day. First, wash your hands with soap and water. Then gently wash the burn and put antibiotic ointment on it. If the burn area is small, a dressing may not be needed during the day. Check the burn every day for signs of infection, such as increased pain, redness, swelling or pus. If you see any of these signs, see your doctor right away. To prevent infection, avoid breaking any blisters that form.

Burned skin itches as it heals. Keep your fingernails cut short and don't scratch the burned skin. The burned area will be sensitive to sunlight for up to one year, so you should apply sunscreen to the area when you're outside.

Third-degree burn

For third-degree burns, go to the hospital right away. Don't take off any clothing that is stuck to the burn. Don't soak the burn in water or apply any ointment. The burned area above the level of the heart. You can cover the burn with a cool, wet sterile bandage or clean cloth until you receive medical assistance.

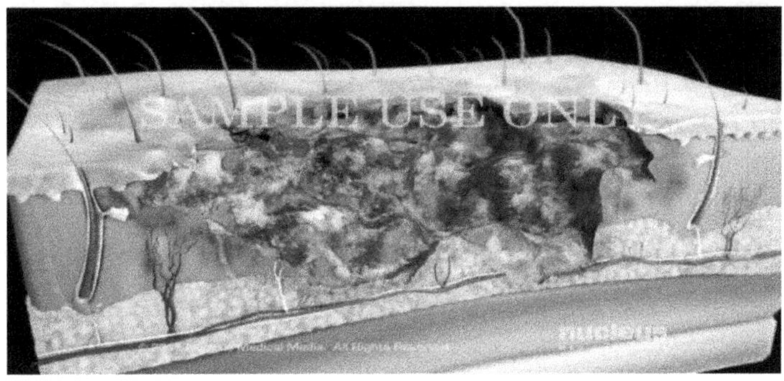

Is there anything I shouldn't do when treating a burn?

Do not put butter or oil on burns. Do not put ice or ice water directly on second- or third-degree burns. If blisters form over the burn, do not break them. These things can cause more damage to the skin.

What do I need to know about electrical and chemical burns?

A person who has an electrical burn (for example, from a power line) should go to the hospital right away. Electrical burns often cause serious injury to organs inside the body. This injury may not show on the skin.

A chemical burn should be flushed with large amounts of cool water. Take off any clothing or jeweler that has the chemical on it. Don't put anything on the burned area, such as antibiotic ointment. This might start a chemical reaction that could make the burn worse. You can wrap the burn with dry, sterile gauze or a clean cloth. If you don't know what to do, call 911 or your local poison control center, or see your doctor right away.

8.3 Fracture

A dislocation is where a bone has been displaced from its normal position at a joint. A fracture is when a bone has been broken.

A fracture is termed: Closed where there is no break in the skin; Open where the bone end has broken the skin or a wound is present with the fracture.

The fractured or dislocated part should not be moved and first aid should be confined to providing soft padding and support in the position chosen by the patient.

In a remote area, or where ambulance or medical care is likely to be delayed for an hour or more, the first aider may use simple immobilization techniques to reduce pain and spasm.

In such cases it is the first aider's responsibility to monitor the circulation in any affected limb to ensure that the immobilization has not stopped blood flow or affected the nerve supply to an extremity.

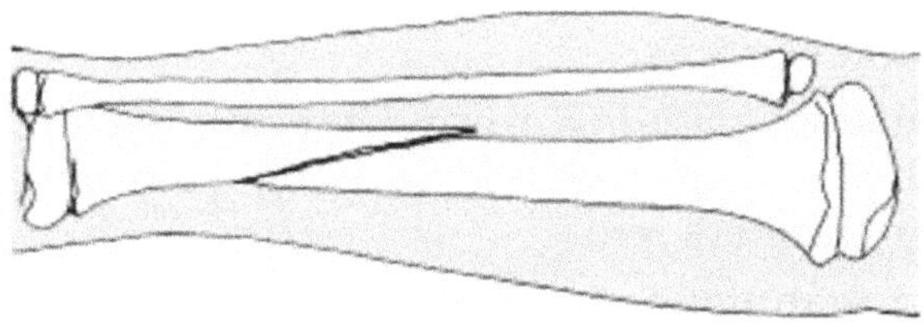

Closed fracture

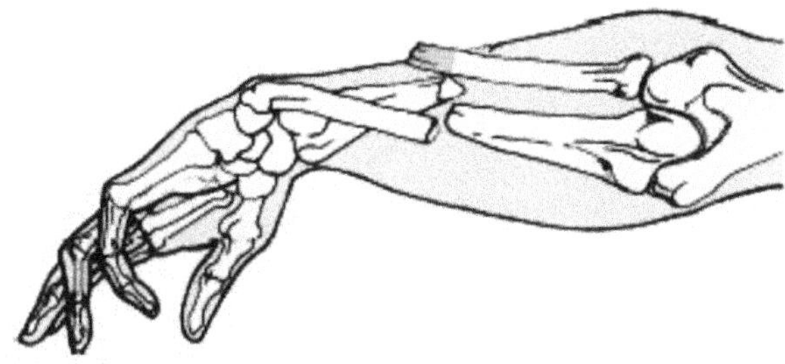

Open fracture

Symptoms and signs – Not all may be present

Pain, swelling, deformity of the injured area (when compared with the uninjured side of the body), loss of normal function of the injured part, discoloration of the skin (i.e. blueness) or bruising a wound if it is an open fracture, altered sensation – e.g. 'pins and needles' – if a nerve is under pressure grating sensation if injured bone ends are rubbing together patient may have heard/felt the bone break

How you can help

1. ***Control any bleeding*:** If a wound is present, check for any significant bleeding; and if bleeding, apply direct pressure around any exposed bones.

   Apply padding around the wound, or above and below the wound. Apply a clean dressing loosely over the injured part.

   Call 108 for an ambulance.

2. ***Immobilize the injured part*:** Reduce the pain and the risk of further injury by supporting and immobilizing the injured area. Usually this simply means supporting the injured part in a comfortable position.

3. ***Make the patient comfortable*:** Help the patient into the position of greatest comfort without any unnecessary

movement. Use blankets, pillows or clothing for general comfort and support.

Place generous padding around the injured area and in the nearby hollows of the body, using soft towels, clothing, pillows or blankets, etc.

Where an ambulance is likely to be delayed for more than 1 hour immobilize the injured part. Specific immobilization techniques for various injuries are outlined on the following pages.

DO NOT move the patient or any injured part unnecessarily.

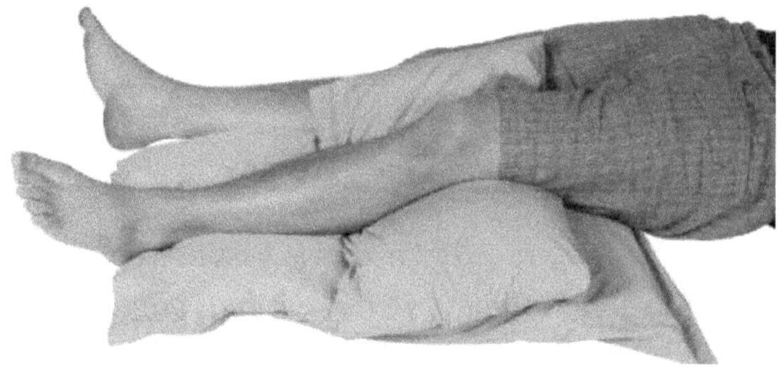

Make the patient comfortable

Fractures and dislocations that need special care

Fracture of the face or jaw

Fractures of the face and jaw have the potential to be serious. Injuries to the face may be associated with a head injury or with a serious eye injury. A fractured or dislocated jaw may cause a risk of serious airway complications because of the loss of the ability to swallow or bleeding within the mouth.

If unconscious but breathing normally, place the patient on their side in a supported position.

Call 108 for an ambulance.

If conscious, allow the patient to rest in the position of greatest comfort, generally half-sitting or lying down with the head tilted to the injured side. Provide a clean pad or some tissues for the patient to mop up any blood, saliva or mucus.

If the jaw appears broken or dislocated, allow the patient to support the injured part with one or both hands. Fracture of the collarbone or dislocation of the shoulder joint

A dislocated shoulder and fractured collarbone are managed in a similar way because both injuries disrupt the shoulder joint, and the weight of the arm on the injured side needs to be supported. Usually the patient will be supporting the arm on the injured side and the shoulder will be lower than the uninjured side, with the patient's head tilted towards the injury. The patient is usually in severe pain and any unnecessary movement should be avoided.

Use a pillow or folded clothing to allow the patient to support the weight of the arm in the most comfortable position.

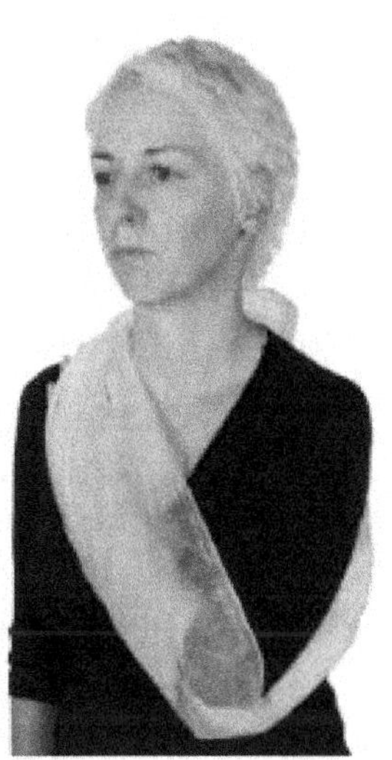

Call 108 for an ambulance.

If ambulance transport is likely to be delayed, carefully immobilize the arm with padding under the armpit and apply either an elevation sling or an arm sling depending on the patient's preferred position of greatest comfort. Use a pillow or folded clothing to allow the patient support the weight of the arm in the most comfortable position. Apply either an elevation sling, or an arm sling.

Fracture of the ribs

The injury may involve a single broken rib or several broken ribs. A rib fracture is always associated with pain, especially when breathing in or coughing. Sometimes an abnormal movement can be seen where one part of the chest moves outwards when the corresponding part on the opposite side moves inwards. In a severe injury where the underlying lung has been damaged, the patient may have breathing

Assist the patient into a position of greatest comfort. Call 108 for an ambulance.

If severe pain is present, the first aider should apply improvised padding over the injured area and a broad-fold triangular bandage as a binder to secure the arm to the chest wall over the padding. This will stabilize the moving segment internal injury. An elevation sling is used to support the arm on the injured side.

Fracture of the upper arm

The patient usually supports the weight of the elbow and lower arm to reduce the pain of the injury. This fracture can be very serious because of the risk of pressure on major nerves and blood vessels, especially those close to the shoulder and elbow joints.

Assist the patient into a position of greatest comfort, generally sitting in a chair or half sitting with support.

Allow the patient to support the arm on the injured side on a pillow or folded clothing.

Call 108 for an ambulance.

If the ambulance is likely to be delayed apply an elevation sling with the minimum of movement of the injured arm.

Fracture of the lower arm or wrist

These injuries are very common, especially in children and the older adult. The wrist is often injured when a person falls onto an outstretched hand. Normally the patient can support the injured arm using the other arm, but additional immobilization may be required during transport to a doctor or hospital.

Assist the patient into the position of greatest comfort, usually sitting down supporting the weight of the injured limb against the body with the other hand. A pillow or rolled-up clothing may be placed on the lap to provide a soft support for the patient to use to rest the weight of the arm.

The patient needs to be taken to a hospital. If ambulance transport is not used it is necessary to immobilize the arm to avoid more pain and muscle spasm.

Apply a splint under the injured limb using firmly rolled newspaper folded into a gutter shape.

Hold the splint in place with a narrow-fold bandage applied above and below the injury site, with an additional bandage if necessary.

Apply an arm sling for additional support and stability.

Fracture of the hand and fracture or dislocation of a finger

Injuries of the hand and fingers are common in some sports. Although it is tempting to replace a dislocated finger to relieve the pain and muscle spasm, there is a risk that a small nerve or blood vessel may be trapped and lead to a permanently numb or 'dead' finger. Replacement should be done only by a doctor or physiotherapist.

Apply generous soft padding around the hand or injured finger(s).

Apply an elevation sling, taking care to avoid touching the hand or fingers when tying the knot.

The patient needs to be taken to a hospital.

Fracture or dislocation of the ankle, foot or toes

It is often difficult to decide whether an ankle joint is fractured or sprained, and whenever there is any doubt, the injury should be managed as a potential fracture. The foot and toes can be crushed by a heavy object, which results in a very painful and disabling injury.

Assist the patient to lie down and try to raise the injured foot and ankle on soft padding as soon as possible to reduce pain and slow the onset of swelling.

Unless you suspect an open wound on the foot or toes, leave a well-fitting shoe in place because removal may further complicate the injury.

8.4 Suffocation

Suffocation is a condition where the oxygen level reduces in the blood with an increase in the carbon dioxide concentration resulting in death or unconsciousness.

1. **The different types of asphyxia are**

   Suffocation by toxic gases.

   Drowning.

   Choking due to the entry of a foreign substance.

   Strangulation.

   Asthma.

   Severe infections of the throat

Artificial respiration

Fetal asphyxia

2. **First aid for Suffocation**

Firstly ensure a patent airway.

Check for the respiratory rate.

Check for the level of cyanosis.

In case of drowning, tilt the client to one side with head down.

If strangulation is the cause then remove the band that is constricting the throat.

Asphyxia caused due to swelling of the throat or asthma make the victim sit upright and ensure fresh air.

In case of suffocation by gases remove the victim as soon as possible to fresh air.

For all the victims loosen the clothing surrounding the neck.

If breathing gets restored give sips of cold water.

If breathing does not restore then start artificial respiration.

The artificial respiration followed is mouth-to-mouth respiration. Follow the procedure given below:

Firstly place the victim on his/her back.

Tilt his head at the back.

Pinch the nostrils.

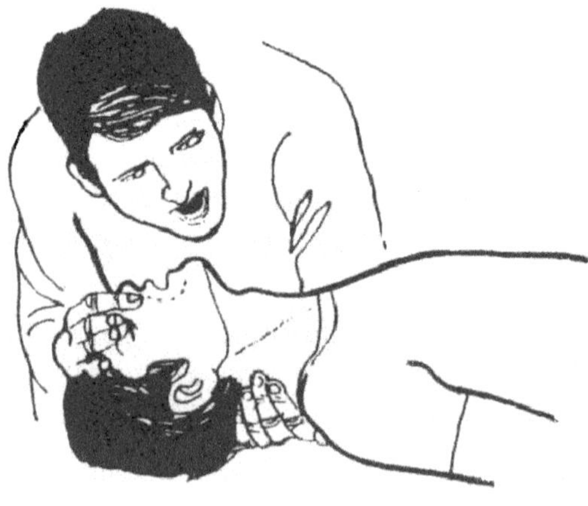

Cover the mouth of the causality.

Blow into his lungs until his chest expands.

Repeat it 15-20 times.

Blowing of air should be done with an open mouth, covering both the mouth and nose.

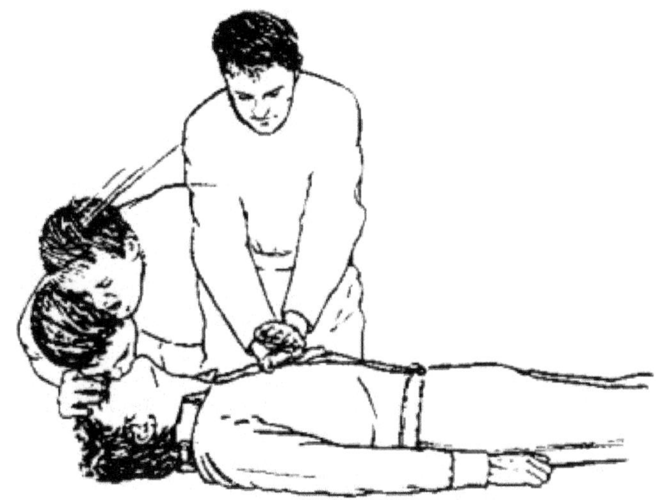

On the other hand, ensure medical help.

If you cannot give two effective breaths, start chest compressions.

The first-aider should give 15chest compressions, then give 2 inflations to the lungs and then again start 15 chest compressions.

The cycle should be continued until the patient recovers or till medical aid is called for.

NOT

When giving chest compressions remember to observe for the following:

Bluish discoloration of the face

Dilated pupils

Pulse rates (Carotid artery)

If the patient recovers, let the victim rest for some time and if he does not recover then call for the medical aid immediately.

8.5 Toxic Ingestion

Poisoning is caused by swallowing, injecting, breathing in, or otherwise being exposed to a harmful substance. Most poisonings occur by accident. Immediate first aid is very important in a poisoning emergency. The first aid you give before getting medical help can save a person's life. This is for information only and not for use in the treatment or management of an actual poison exposure.

Considerations

Millions of poisonings are reported to Indian poison control centers every year, with many deaths. It is important to note that just because a package does not have a warning label doesn't mean it is safe. You should consider poisoning if someone suddenly becomes sick for no apparent reason, or if the person is found near a furnace, car, fire, or in an area that is not well ventilated.

Symptoms of poisoning may take time to develop. However, if you think someone has been poisoned, do not wait for symptoms to develop before getting that person medical help.

Causes

Items that can cause poisoning include:

Carbon monoxide gas (from furnaces, gas engines, fires, space heaters)

Certain foods

Chemicals in the workplace

Drugs, including over-the-counter and prescription medicines (such as an aspirin overdose) and illicit drugs such as cocaine

Household detergents and cleaning products

Household and outdoor plants (eating toxic plants)

Insecticides

Paints

Symptoms

Symptoms vary according to the poison, but may include:

Abdominal pain, Bluish lips, Chest pain, Confusion, Cough, Diarrhea, Difficulty breathing or shortness of breath, Dizziness,

Double vision, Drowsiness, Fever, Headache, Heart palpitations, Irritability, Loss of appetite, Loss of bladder control, Muscle twitching, Nausea and vomiting, Numbness and tingling, Seizures, Skin rash or burns, Stupor, Unconsciousness, Unusual breath odor, Weakness, First Aid, Seek immediate medical help.

For poisoning by swallowing

Check and monitor the person's airway, breathing, and pulse. If necessary, begin rescue breathing and CPR.

Try to make sure that the person has indeed been poisoned. It may be hard to tell. Some signs include chemical-smelling breath, burns around the mouth, difficulty breathing, vomiting, or unusual odors on the person. If possible, identify the poison.

Do NOT make a person throw up unless told to do so by poison control or a health care professional.

If the person vomits, clear the person's airway. Wrap a cloth around your fingers before cleaning out the mouth and throat. If the person has been sick from a plant part, save the vomit. It may help experts identify what medicine can be used to help reverse the poisoning.

If the person starts having convulsions, give convulsion first aid.

Keep the person comfortable. The person should be rolled onto the left side, and remain there while getting or waiting for medical help.

If the poison has spilled on the person's clothes, remove the clothing and flush the skin with water.

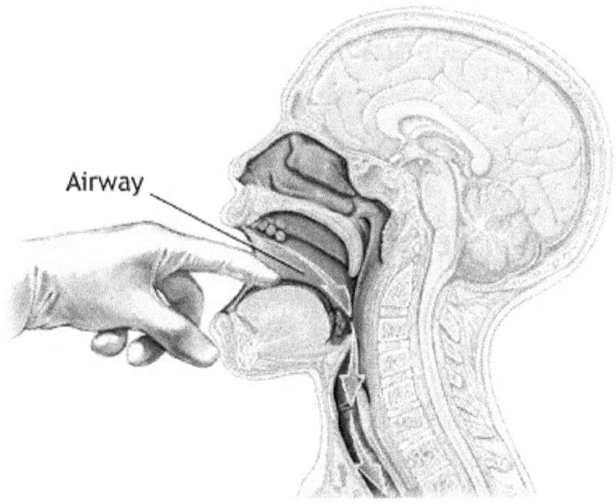

For inhalation poisoning

Call for emergency help. Never attempt to rescue a person without notifying others first.

If it is safe to do so, rescue the person from the danger of the gas, fumes, or smoke. Open windows and doors to remove the fumes.

Take several deep breaths of fresh air, and then hold your breath as you go in. Hold a wet cloth over your nose and mouth.

Do not light a match or use a lighter because some gases can catch fire.

After rescuing the person from danger, check and monitor the person's airway, breathing, and pulse. If necessary, begin rescue breathing and CPR.

If necessary, perform first aid for eye injuries or convulsion first aid.

If the person vomits, clear the person's airway. Wrap a cloth around your fingers before cleaning out the mouth and throat.

Even if the person seems perfectly fine, get medical help.

DO NOT

Do not give an unconscious person anything by mouth.

Do not induce vomiting unless you are told to do so by the Poison Control Center or a doctor. A strong poison that burns on the way down the throat will also do damage on the way back up.

Do not try to neutralize the poison with lemon juice or vinegar, or any other substance, unless you are told to do so by the Poison Control Center or a doctor.

Do not use any "cure-all" type antidote.

Do not wait for symptoms to develop if you suspect that someone has been poisoned.

Prevention

Be aware of poisons in and around your home. Take steps to protect young children from toxic substances. Store all medicines, cleaners, cosmetics, and household chemicals out of reach of children, or in cabinets with childproof latches.

Be familiar with plants in your home, yard, and vicinity. Keep your children informed, too. Remove any poisonous plants. Never eat wild plants, mushrooms, roots, or berries unless you very familiar with them.

Teach children about the dangers of substances that contain poison. Label all poisons.

Don't store household chemicals in food containers, even if they are labeled. Most nonfood substances are poisonous if taken in large doses.

If you are concerned that industrial poisons might be polluting nearby land or water, report your concerns to the local health department or the state or federal Environmental Protection Agency.

8.6 Bleeding Wounds

Bleeding is severe

You suspect internal bleeding

There is an abdominal or chest wound

Bleeding can't be stopped after 10 minutes of firm and steady pressure

Blood spurts out of wound

Stop Bleeding

Apply direct pressure on the cut or wound with a clean cloth, tissue, or piece of gauze until bleeding stops.

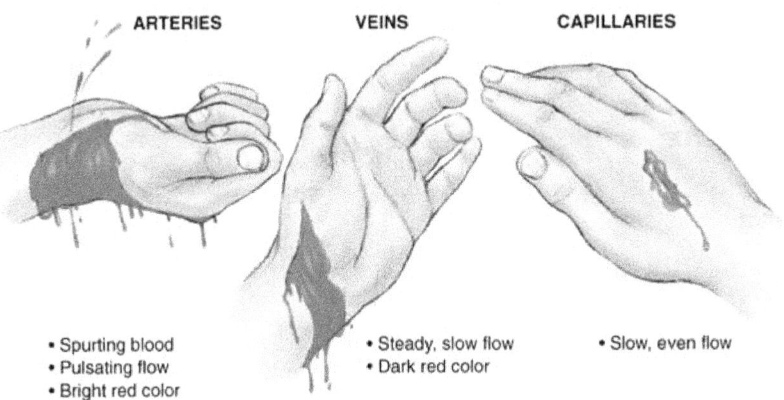

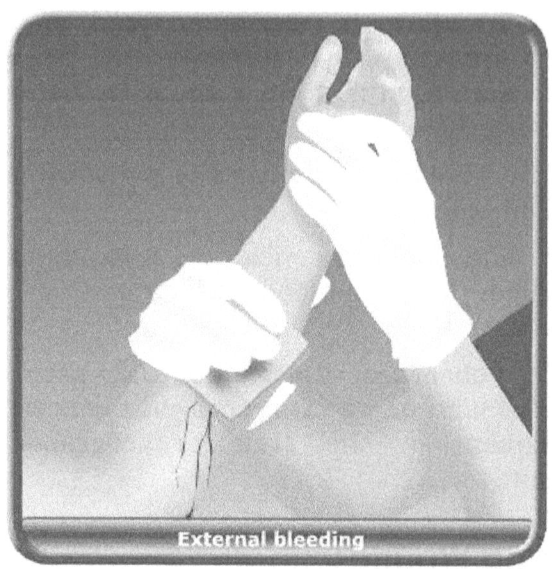

External bleeding

If blood soaks through the material, don't remove it. Put more cloth or gauze on top of it and continue to apply pressure.

If the wound is on the arm or leg, raise limb above the heart to help slow bleeding.

Wash your hands again after giving first aid and before cleaning and dressing the wound.

Do not apply a tourniquet unless the bleeding is severe and not stopped with direct pressure.

Clean Cut or Wound

Gently clean with soap and warm water. Try to rinse soap out of wound to prevent irritation.

Don't use hydrogen peroxide or iodine, which can damage tissue.

Protect the Wound

Apply antibiotic cream to reduce risk of infection and cover with a sterile bandage.

Change the bandage daily to keep the wound clean and dry.

When to Call a Doctor

The wound is deep or the edges are jagged or gaping open.

The wound is on the person's face.

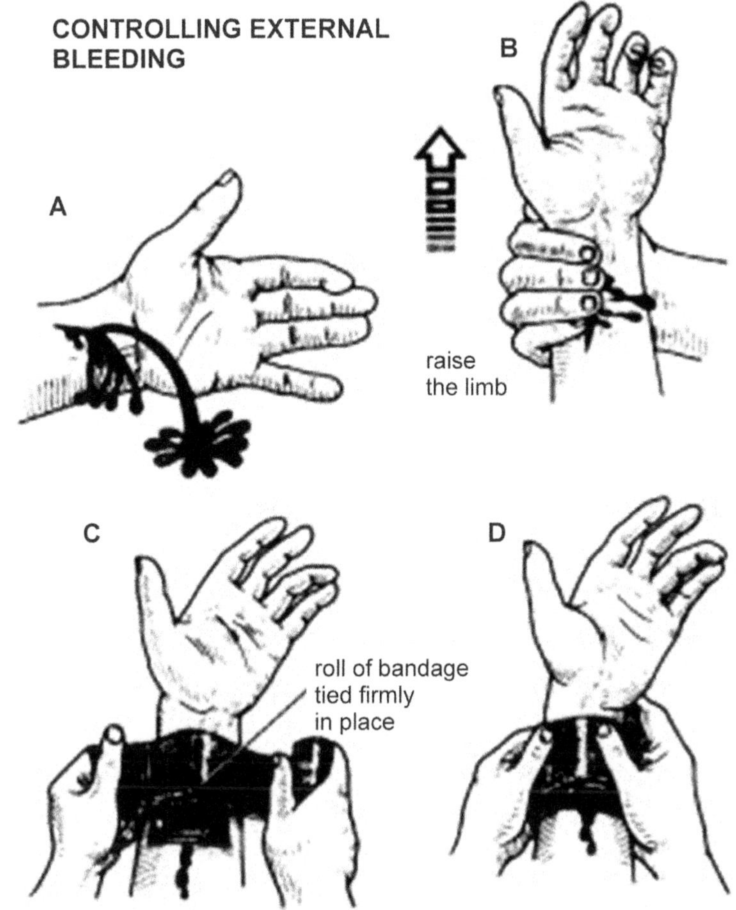

The wound has dirt or debris that won't come out.

The wound shows signs of infection, such as redness, tenderness, or a thick discharge, or if the person runs a temperature over 100° F.

The area around the wound feels numb.

Red streaks form around the wound.

The person has a puncture wound or deep cut and hasn't had a tetanus shot in the past five years, or anyone who hasn't had a tetanus shot in the past 10 years.

Nosebleeds Treatment

Have the person sit up straight and lean forward slightly. Don't have the person lie down or tilt the head backward.

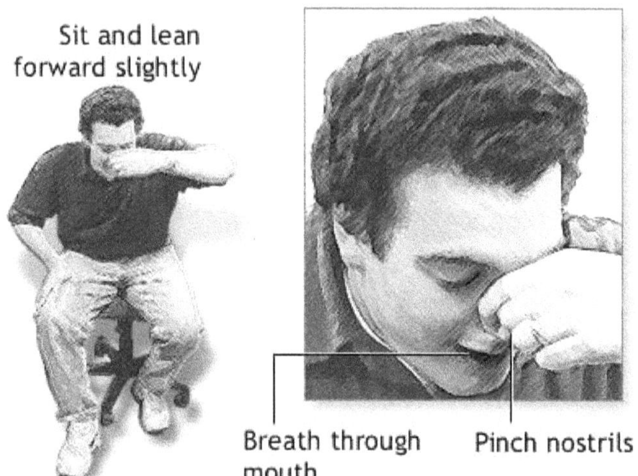

With thumb and index finger, firmly pinch the nose just below the bone up against the face.

Apply pressure for 5 minutes. Time yourself with a clock.

If bleeding continues after 5 minutes, repeat the process.

1. ***Call a Health Care Provider***: See a health care provider immediately if:

   Nosebleed doesn't stop after 10 minutes of home treatment

   The person is taking blood thinners, such as warfarin (Coumadin) or aspirin, or has a bleeding disorder

   Nosebleed happens after a severe head injury or a blow to the face

2. ***Medical Treatment***: The health care provider may use specialized cotton material, insert a balloon in the nose, or use a special electrical tool to cauterize the blood vessels.

3. ***Follow Up***: Broken noses often are not fixed immediately. The care provider will refer the person to a specialist for a consultation once the swelling goes down.

The person should avoid strenuous activity; bending over; and blowing, rubbing or picking the nose until it heals.

8.7 Artificial Respiration

It is clearly specified about artificial in 8.4 Suffocation.

8.8 Cardio-Pulmonary Resuscitation (CPR)

Cardiopulmonary resuscitation (CPR) is the name for a number of procedures that should be applied if a person stop breathing, or if they suffered from cardiac arrest. These measures are performed to keep up an artificial circulation, so that vital organs still get oxygen. CPR does not start a person's heart again, but it can keep the blood (which carries oxygen) flowing around the body long enough for proper emergency treatment to be given.

CPR can be done at different levels. People outside the medical profession are usually expected to recognize the condition, to alert emergency services, and to keep up the artificial respiration, perhaps with the use of an automated tool, called defibrillator. Emergency staff is trained to restart the circulation, and to get the patient's heart beating again. These people can use drugs, intubation, artificial pacemakers and defibrillation to achieve this result.

CPR is normally started on a person who is not breathing and is unconscious. It is continued until the heart can be restarted or the cause is diagnosed. CPR consists of regular compressions (pressing down) of the chest and rescue breathing. If a person's heart is working properly but they are not breathing, the aided breathing is called artificial respiration.

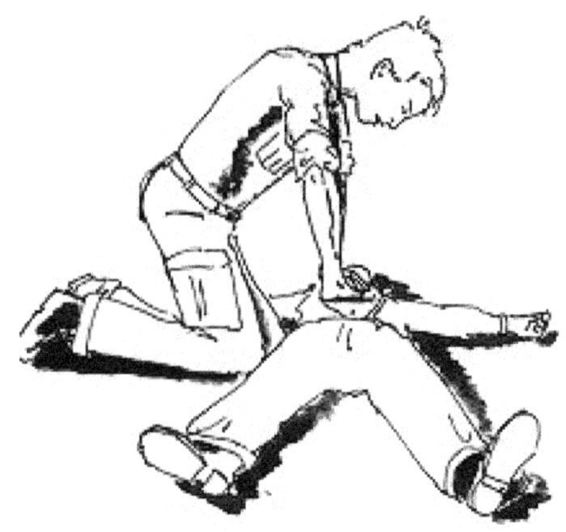

The aim of CPR is to keep a small amount of oxygenated blood flowing to the brain and heart so that, if they are successfully resuscitated, they are not permanently brain damaged.

Statistics

Time is a very important factor. Each minute that passes before the onset of the CPR measures lowers the chance of survival by about ten percent. In the case where the CPR starts within the first three to five minutes, and a defibrillator is available, the chance of survival can be as high as 50, or even 75% (That is: one out of two, or one out of four not surviving). In European countries, emergency services take about eight minutes or more to arrive, once they have been alerted. A victim's survival therefore largely depends on the presence and quick action of other people present. A quick call to emergency services, and a quick start of basic CPR, especially fibrillation can double to triple the chance of survival with adults, and children.

How to survive a heart attack alone?

Since many people are alone when they suffer a heart attack. The person whose heart is beating improperly begins to feel faint and has only 10 seconds left before losing consciousness.

However these victims can help themselves by coughing repeatedly and very vigorously. A deep breadth should be taken before each cough, and the cough must be deep and prolonged, as when producing sputum from deep inside the chest. A breadth and a cough must be repeated about every 2 seconds without let up until help arrives or until the heart is felt to be beating normally again.

Deep breadths get oxygen into the lungs and coughing movements squeeze the heart and keep the blood circulating. The squeezing pressure on the heart also helps to regain normal rhythm. In this way the heart attack victims can get to a hospital after the event.

www.ingramcontent.com/pod-product-compliance
Ingram Content Group UK Ltd.
Pitfield, Milton Keynes, MK11 3LW, UK
UKHW021830190726
13853UKWH00003B/1274